THE
ALZHEIMER'S
FAMILY

THE ALZHEIMER'S FAMILY

Helping Caregivers Cope

ROBERT B. SANTULLI, MD

W. W. Norton & Company
New York • London

For information about permission to reproduce selections from this book, write to
Permissions, W. W. Norton & Company, Inc., 500 Fifth Avenue, New York, NY 10110

For information about special discounts for bulk purchases, please contact W. W. Norton
Special Sales at specialsales@wwnorton.com or 800-233-4830

Manufacturing by RR Donnelley, Bloomsburg
Book design by Bytheway Publishing Services
Production manager: Leeann Graham

Library of Congress Cataloging-in-Publication Data

Santulli, Robert B.
    The Alzheimer's family : helping caregivers cope / Robert B. Santulli.—1st ed.
        p. ; cm.
    "A Norton professional book"
    Includes bibliographical references and index.
    ISBN 978-0-393-70577-5 (hardcover)
    1. Alzheimer's disease—Patients—Care.   2. Alzheimer's disease—Patients—Family
relationships.   3. Caregivers—Psychology.   I. Title.
    [DNLM: 1. Alzheimer Disease—nursing.   2. Alzheimer Disease—psychology.
3. Caregivers—psychology.   4. Family Relations.   WM 155]
    RC523.S275 2011
    362.196'831—dc22   2011010951

ISBN: 978-0-393-70577-5

W. W. Norton & Company, Inc., 500 Fifth Avenue, New York, N.Y. 10110
www.wwnorton.com
W. W. Norton & Company Ltd., Castle House, 75/76 Wells Street, London W1T 3QT

1 2 3 4 5 6 7 8 9 0

To my family: Linda, Stephen, and Elizabeth

"The family is one of nature's masterpieces."
—George Santayana

CONTENTS

ACKNOWLEDGMENTS

Many people have been extremely helpful to me in creating this volume. First, I would like to thank Charles (Andy) Anderson, whose generous donation in memory of his wife spawned the creation at Dartmouth of The Jeanne Estee Mackay Anderson Alzheimer's Disease Support and Education Fund. The Anderson Fund has given me the opportunity to focus my work more comprehensively on the needs of the Alzheimer's family. This book is a direct result of that opportunity.

I would like to thank Caroline Moore and the rest of her staff at the Dartmouth-Hitchcock Aging Resource Center. They have been wonderful colleagues and aids throughout this process. They have also become an invaluable presence for Alzheimer's families throughout New Hampshire and Vermont.

I would also like to thank Kesstan Blandin, PhD, the Upper Valley Program Coordinator for the Alzheimer's Association of Massachusetts and New Hampshire. Dr. Blandin's intelligence, kindness, and tireless work with Alzheimer's families have been a source of wonderful inspiration and valuable learning for me.

In addition, I wish to thank Erin Onstad, a graduate student at the Dartmouth Institute for Health Policy and Clinical Practice, for her assistance with issues related to Alzheimer's care in the assisted living setting.

I have learned much about Alzheimer's disease from medical texts and scholarly articles, and from conferences, seminars, lectures, and other professional educational resources. But my most valuable learning, by far, has come from the many Alzheimer's individuals and families I have had the privilege of knowing over the past four decades. I have cared for many of these in my clinical practice; others have attended the various Alzheimer's support groups I have facilitated. We have struggled together with the many difficult issues that arise in this terrible disease. Mere words cannot convey how thankful I am to those Alzheimer's families who taught me so much—not only about the disease and its impact on families, but about the enormous strength of the human spirit in the face of terrible adversity.

I would also like to thank Andrea Costella Dawson, Vani Kannan, Karen Fisher, and the rest of the editorial staff at Norton who helped get my ideas into an organized, readable, and hopefully useful format. In particular, Andrea Costella Dawson's wisdom and intelligence have been outstanding, surpassed only by her patience and tolerance when, all too often, other professional activities pushed this work to the side.

Finally, there were many weekends when my involvement with *The Alzheimer's Family* competed with my involvement with my own family. I want to thank them, again, for their forbearance. We are all glad for the completion of this volume. I do hope it will be interesting, informative and useful. Although I have emphasized how many different people have been helpful along the way, I am solely responsible for any errors of commission or omission.

THE
ALZHEIMER'S
FAMILY

INTRODUCTION

ALZHEIMER'S:
THE DISEASE OF THE 21ST CENTURY

A generation ago, cancer was looked upon with great fear, as an incurable death sentence. People talked about it in hushed tones, afraid to utter the "C word" because of the extreme reactions it produced. While cancer is still dreaded, there has been much progress in its treatment, and some forms of cancer are now seen as a chronic illness to be managed. Along with significant advances in care, the stigma associated with the disease has declined, and the condition is much more openly discussed in the public arena.

In the 1980s, AIDS began to replace cancer as the most feared disease in the minds of many. To a great degree, this had to do with the lack of effective treatments initially, and it was—accurately—seen as inevitably fatal. AIDS (like most cancers, certainly) remains an extremely serious condition, of course, but as effective treatments have been developed, some of the extreme fears of the disease and the stigma associated with it have begun to lessen.

Now, it would appear that Alzheimer's disease is becoming the illness that people—particularly those at or beyond middle age—fear the most.

Although Alzheimer's disease can occur earlier in life, it is primarily a disease of the aged. Overall, about 13% of persons over age 65 have Alzheimer's disease. At age 65, however, only about 2% suffer from the illness. However, every 5 years, the percentage of persons with the disease doubles, so that by 70, nearly 5% have it; at 75, about 10% of the population, and at 80, at least 20%. By 85, some 40% of those still living meet criteria for Alzheimer's disease (Alzheimer's Association, 2011).

Males and females seem to be affected at approximately the same rate, but since a greater number of older females are alive than males, more women than men are living with the disease. According to *The Shriver Report: A Woman's Nation Takes on Alzheimer's* (2010) about two thirds of people with Alzheimer's disease are women. And women comprise about 60% of the caregivers.

Alzheimer's disease is a type of dementia (about which more later); it is the most common cause of dementia by far. According to some studies, Alzheimer's disease, by itself or in combination with another form of dementia, accounts for as much as 75% of all cases of dementing illness. However, other forms of dementia often present very similar issues to the family, in terms of the nature of symptoms and the effects on the caregiver. In many ways, from the caregiver's perspective, there may be more similarities than differences among the different forms of dementia. Thus, while this book primarily concerns the Alzheimer's family, much of the content is also relevant to family members of people with other types of dementia. Other common dementias include the following:

- Vascular dementia
- Mixed dementia
- Dementia with Lewy bodies
- Dementia of Parkinson's disease
- Frontotemporal dementia

For simplicity's sake, and because it covers the vast majority of persons with dementia, the primary caregiver and other family members of the patient are referred to as "the Alzheimer's family," but in many cases the phrase "the dementia family" might be an appropriate substitute.

While most people with Alzheimer's develop the illness in late life (the late 60s and older), it can begin much earlier, in the 40s, 50s, or early 60s. Fortunately, this is uncommon—less than 4% of those with Alzheimer's disease have early onset (starting before age 65). Having early-onset Alzheimer's disease adds another level of tragedy and an even greater burden to the person with the disease, and the family. While this book primarily addresses the issues surrounding Alzheimer's that begins in later life, much of it applies to early-onset families as well.

A GROWING CRISIS AS THE POPULATION AGES

Alzheimer's disease is a growing crisis. As the baby boomers—that large cohort of individuals born in the years immediately following World War II—enter their 60s, in the coming decades the numbers of persons with the disease will increase significantly. It is estimated that, if no cure or prevention is developed, 13–15 million people will have the disease by 2050, due to the increased numbers of elders in the population (Alzheimer's Association, 2011). Worldwide this is true as well, and numbers of cases are rising most rapidly in developing countries, which have the fewest resources to care for those with the disease. This is not because Alzheimer's is spreading like a virus or other communicable disease, but simply because there are increasing numbers of older people with each passing year.

The diagnosis of Alzheimer's disease is often considerably delayed, for a variety of reasons, including the gradual onset of the disease, the subtle nature of the early symptoms, and the time and expertise it takes for a busy physician to take the history and perform the necessary office tests. In addition, the stigma surrounding the disease and denial on the part of the individual and family can significantly delay diagnosis. However, delaying a diagnostic evaluation for a significant period of time after the onset of symptoms means that the family and patient are subjected to a great deal of unnecessary stress and uncertainty about what is wrong with the individual who is becoming deeply forgetful, having greater and greater difficulties functioning, and perhaps having significant changes of personality. This "pre-diagnostic" phase of the illness is usually extremely difficult for the person with the disease and for the family. Many questions go unanswered; blame and anger are often plentiful; and increasingly dangerous behaviors can occur. Delaying diagnosis delays the opportunity for families to plan for their future based on knowing what lies ahead. Finally, a significant delay in diagnosis means that pharmacologic treatment gets put off until a great deal more irreversible damage has occurred. While our current medication treatments for Alzheimer's disease are modestly effective, at best, it does seem clear that starting treatment earlier in the disease leads to better outcomes rather than waiting unnecessarily.

Once a diagnosis is finally made, patients and family members generally feel a deep sense of sadness and a variety of other unpleasant emotions, of course; but there is often a feeling of relief, as well, now that they know what they are dealing with. The anxiety surrounding the symptoms actually goes down once a diagnosis has been made.

When one person has Alzheimer's disease, many are affected. According to the Alzheimer's Association, for every person with the disease, at least four individuals' lives are deeply touched by the illness. Usually there is a primary caregiver, often a spouse or an adult child, who bears the major responsibility of caring for the individual with the disease. However, other caregivers are frequently involved also—as well there should be: this is too big a job for just one person. Whether or not other family members play a significant role in providing assistance or monitoring for the person with Alzheimer's, all family members are involved and affected to a greater or lesser degree, including the nuclear family and often the extended family as well. It includes those who live with the patient, those who live nearby, and even those who live some distance away. Alzheimer's stresses the entire family. This disease can bring into bold relief the enormous strengths of families when confronted with a crisis. However, it can also bring to the surface vulnerabilities and unresolved conflicts—problems that tend to be ignored or avoided when there are no crises. The disease and its stresses can even tear a family apart. Such outcomes are not rare and immeasurably increase the tragedy of the disease itself.

FAMILY: THE CRITICAL LINK

As difficult as it can be for family members to cope with a loved one with Alzheimer's disease, family members are also the most critical component, by far, in the network of care for the person with Alzheimer's. It is clear that caregivers and other family members who are very knowledgeable about the illness, who understand and have come to terms with their own emotional reactions to the situation, who feel understood and supported in their caregiving decisions, and who have learned to effectively balance the needs of the person with Alzheimer's on the one hand, and their own needs on the other, will cope with this overwhelming task much more effectively. They have a greater sense of emotional well-being, feel less burdened, and have an enhanced ability to continue the process without becoming demoralized or burned out. Frequently, this leads to the loved one with Alzheimer's doing significantly better in a number of important domains, as well.

A CLINICIAN FOR THE PRIMARY CAREGIVER AND OTHER FAMILY MEMBERS

Someone who has Alzheimer's disease needs to be cared for by a physician who is expert in making the diagnosis and treating the disease and the various complications throughout its course. Likewise, the Alzheimer's family—the primary caregiver and other family members who are involved—will benefit enormously from the opportunity to work with someone who understands the profound impact of this disease on the family, and the impact of the family on the person with the disease, and can serve as a guide and aide throughout this very difficult journey. This volume has been written for such professionals. Throughout this book, these health care professionals are referred to simply as *clinicians*. This includes physicians, psychologists, social workers, psychotherapists, counselors, care managers, case workers, nurse practitioners, and the staff of senior centers, senior care agencies, and long-term care facilities.

It is hoped that this volume will help these clinicians better understand the impact of the disease on the family, and the impact of the family on the disease. It should give clinicians the tools they need to help families cope more effectively, for their own health and emotional well-being, and for the sake of the person with the disease. It will help clinicians understand the unique stresses faced by members of the Alzheimer's family. It provides a great deal of information about the disease itself and what particular challenges to expect in the various stages of the illness. It suggests therapeutic approaches and other strategies for addressing these issues in ways that will help family members understand and cope with the symptoms and behaviors of the patient, as well as to understand and cope more effectively with their own emotional and psychological reactions to this difficult situation. In addition, it will help clinicians to identify and treat family members who are especially distressed by the disease and to be helpful in cases where the disease has created (or brought to the surface) family conflicts and disagreements that add significant additional stresses. Well-informed clinicians can also assist with some of the difficult decisions that regularly arise in the care of persons with Alzheimer's.

How, exactly, do these clinicians become involved in caring for family members of persons with Alzheimer's disease? In some cases, a clinician may already be caring for the person with the disease, and recognizes the importance of helping the family as well, for their own sake and the sake of the patient. In other cases, a clinician may be working with someone whose family member has just been diagnosed with Alzheimer's disease. A clinician may work in a practice setting in which the person with Alzheimer's disease is treated primarily by a neurologist or other physician, and family members are routinely or selectively seen by another (often non-MD) clinician on the team. Or a family member may independently, or by referral, seek treatment from the clinician to get help in coping with this disease in a loved one.

However the connection is made, it is increasingly common that clinicians are called upon to work with family members of Alzheimer's patients. And because of the enormous impact of the disease on the caregiver, and the equally great impact of the caregiver on the person with Alzheimer's, it is critical that clinicians working with family members have a thorough understanding of the disease and the myriad ways in which family members are entwined in it.

Alzheimer's disease is a long and difficult journey. Family members who are unfortunate enough to have to take this journey do need a guiding hand through the process. It is hoped that this book will provide clinicians with the information and the tools they need to effectively serve in that role.

CHAPTER 1

The Alzheimer's Family

UNDERSTANDING THE ALZHEIMER'S FAMILY

Alzheimer's disease is, indeed, a family illness. Just as the illness affects individuals differently, depending on many factors including their premorbid personality or character, the disease affects families in different ways depending, to a great degree, on the *character* of the family. To understand the impact of the disease on a particular family, it is critical to have a good understanding of their dynamics. It is important to know, for example, what the power relationships in the family were before the person became ill. For example, has there been a great deal of mutuality between husband and wife, or did one tend to dominate the other? When the dominant member of a couple is the one to develop the disease, difficulties are almost inevitable, as it becomes harder and harder to dominate when one is demented. The dominated spouse has almost always been harboring resentments about this issue, and those resentments tend to come to the surface one way or another, once the illness has developed, if they haven't before that point. One of the first tasks of the clinician working with a member of the Alzheimer's family is to learn as much as possible about the relationship prior to the illness.

Couples who have not talked with each other a great deal about their feelings during their marriage are less likely to openly discuss the illness and its impact on both of them, although this is vital in coping with it, for both the victim and the spouse. Overall, it is probably obvious that couples in a strong, mutual relationship with good communication cope with this illness (and probably most other adversities) better than those who do not have such a solid foundation.

TASKS OF THE PRIMARY CAREGIVER

In most situations, a single individual is designated (officially or unofficially) as the primary caregiver. When there is a living and cognitively capable spouse, the primary caregiver is nearly always this person. Many seniors feel it is their obligation to care for a spouse, no matter how difficult the task might be, and do not want their adult children to be burdened with it. Also, some spouses (or other primary caregivers, for that matter) do not let others help because they want to remain in complete control of the situation. This inevitably creates tension with other family members. And there are times when the spouse does not take very active control of the situation and another family member needs to take over.

It often seems that a disproportionate amount of the work of caregiving falls onto the shoulders of the primary caregiver, while other available family members are often much less involved. This can create a difficult situation for all concerned. In general, the most effective caregiving situations are those in which the primary caregiver has extensive, regular assistance from others, welcoming the help without ambivalence when it is available. The primary caregiver may perform the majority of the tasks, but has regular periods off duty, when others care for the person with Alzheimer's. Indeed, the best outcomes occur when caregiving is a responsibility shared among several family members, all of whom willingly participate in the tasks of care.

What is caregiving? For purposes of this volume, caregiving is defined as all of the activities someone does to supervise or assist the individual with Alzheimer's disease. What are the typical tasks involved in caring for someone with Alzheimer's disease? To a great degree, this varies with the stage of illness and from person to person as well. Nevertheless, it is useful to consider four different categories of providing care to the person with Alzheimer's:

- Passive caregiving
- Active caregiving
- Cognitive caregiving
- Behavioral caregiving

Naturally, these tasks overlap considerably, but I discuss them as separate entities.

Passive Caregiving

Passive caregiving refers to the need to simply be present in case help is needed. In mild Alzheimer's disease, this is less extensive than later in the disease. There is also great variability in how much caregivers feel the need to provide passive caregiving at different stages of the disease. Some caregivers are comfortable leaving the person with early Alzheimer's alone for extended periods, while others feel the need to be with the afflicted individual nearly all of the time. In addition to the general severity of illness, this difference may also have to do with the specific behavior patterns of the person with Alzheimer's. Some people with the disease have significant apathy and are content to sit (or nap) for long periods of time, with little activity or contact with others. While this behavioral pattern can be upsetting to families, particularly in someone who had previously been quite active, these individuals may require less passive caregiving than others who are more active and feel a greater need for contact with the caregiver. A caregiver who is providing passive caregiving may actually do very little for the person with Alzheimer's but needs to be nearby.

For some spousal caregivers, passive caregiving is not especially stressful, as it does not require any great change in the relationship. This is particularly true for older couples who do nearly everything together (even before Alzheimer's), and seem to be almost joined at the hip. However, for most caregivers, particularly those who are not spouses, the need to provide increasing amounts of passive caregiving as the disease progresses is difficult indeed. These caregivers regularly complain of feeling tied down or trapped by the situation. It is all too easy for a caregiver to become resentful toward the person with Alzheimer's for this. The clinician can help caregivers recognize that it is the illness which demands so much from the caregiver, and not the loved one. This may seem obvious in the abstract, but of course it is not always so easy in practice. Clinicians should keep the refrain "blame the disease, not the person" in mind and use it frequently.

As the disease progresses, of course, the need for passive caregiving increases; it becomes less and less desirable or even possible to leave the person alone even for short periods of time. Also, passive caregiving is only passive until the person with Alzheimer's has a need, at which time active caregiving is required. While it is possible to separate active and passive caregiving for the purposes of discussion, in reality caregivers spend their time providing a blend of both passive and active caregiving, in different proportions, depending on the person, on the stage of illness, and other factors.

Active Caregiving

Active caregiving can be further subdivided into (1) role assumption and (2) assistance with specific tasks.

Role Assumption

Role assumption includes taking over those tasks, or roles, which the person with Alzheimer's previously performed but is no longer able to do because of this illness. Most of these tasks are the so-called instrumental activities of daily living, or IADLs:

- Paying the bills and balancing the checkbook
- Cooking
- Doing minor household repairs
- Shopping
- Operating mechanical equipment such as the microwave or the computer

• Taking medications as prescribed
• Driving

Whether or not it is advisable or safe for a person with Alzheimer's disease to continue to drive is often very contentious. This subject is discussed in more detail in Chapter 6. As people with Alzheimer's disease are in the process of losing their ability to perform IADLs, they usually require assistance with these tasks to accomplish them. While it may seem that it would be a simple matter to assist someone with a task, that is often not the case. Needing to be in control is a common trait among people in general; not everyone feels it to a great degree, but of course for some it is extremely important to stay in charge, no matter what. This is seen more commonly (but certainly not exclusively) in males, and in particular among people whose careers or lifestyles have involved being in positions of power over others—executives, career military officers, shop foremen, physicians, and the like. Generally, the degree to which someone needs to be in control does not lessen when that person develops Alzheimer's disease; it can even seem greater than before as the individual struggles with the ability to remain in charge. Adapting to the disease, which inevitably involves yielding control of many things, certainly can be challenging. "Control freaks" have a very difficult time with this aspect of the illness. While he or she may need assistance with a given instrumental task, a person with Alzheimer's who needs to be in control rarely recognizes or acknowledges this. As a result, it can be quite difficult for a caregiver to assist with necessary tasks without causing a great deal of tension. It is important to recognize, as well, that while an intense need for control may not be a very helpful or attractive personality feature in someone who has Alzheimer's, it is usually central to the individual's sense of self-esteem. This may be why those with Alzheimer's who have a high need for control do not give it up without a great struggle. It is not only viewed as an assault on their autonomy but, more basically, it is felt as an attack on a critical component of their self-esteem.

One of the major challenges of caring for someone with Alzheimer's is to find a way to provide increasing amounts of assistance and direction without making the afflicted person feel diminished in the process. This is no easy task; the self-esteem of people with Alzheimer's disease tends to be very fragile. Even (perhaps especially) those who insist that nothing is wrong with them are usually, on some level, aware that they are not functioning normally. They may be not only very defensive about it, but on a deeper level are often anxious, distressed, and feeling very vulnerable about the changes in mental functioning they have experienced. They may be very unlikely to acknowledge these feelings (indeed, they may have no conscious awareness of them) but do need to be treated with this significant vulnerability in mind.

Individuals may finally give up their attempt to remain in control of a given activity when they are no longer able to manage any aspects of the task. At that point, it may become easier for the caregiver to simply assume full management of the task, but with control-oriented persons, this point is usually reached only after some difficult struggles.

Assisting With Specific Tasks

Assisting with or taking over specific tasks is the other form of active caregiving. As the disease progresses, people with Alzheimer's need increasing amounts of assistance not only with IADLs, as discussed above, but also with basic activities of daily living (ADLs):

- Dressing
- Bathing
- Toileting
- Feeding
- Walking

Usually, persons with Alzheimer's lose the ability to perform these tasks independently after several years of illness, but there can be great variability. Needing assistance with basic ADLs usually means that a person has progressed to the moderate stages of illness. The loss of function and consequent need for assistance is usually gradual. For example, someone with Alzheimer's disease may gradually lose the ability to select appropriate items of clothing to wear and the caregiver then needs to assist by making suggestions about this. This will progress to the caregiver needing to lay out all of the clothes for the person to wear. As time goes on, assistance with buttons, zippers, and getting items like shirts and pants on correctly becomes more and more necessary. Finally, the person with Alzheimer's may lose all ability to put on clothing, and the caregiver needs to dress the person entirely.

Many caregivers, particularly elderly spouses, find the physical aspects of caregiving quite challenging, and if they do not have assistance from other family members or paid helpers, need to arrange for it by this stage of the illness. Bladder and, especially, bowel incontinence are extremely difficult for all caregivers to manage. Bowel incontinence is often a last straw that leads a caregiver to consider placing a loved one in long-term care.

Cognitive Caregiving

The third type of caregiving, cognitive care, involves the caregiver serving as an external source of memory and other cognitive functions of the person with Alzheimer's disease. Since short-term memory impairment is one of the earliest and most fundamental symptoms of Alzheimer's, this form of caregiving generally begins earlier than passive or active caregiving and continues, increasingly, throughout the disease. It usually begins even before the individual has a diagnosis—sometimes long before. Most individuals with mild cognitive impairment (often a pre-Alzheimer's condition that involves deficits in recent memory but no major impairment in any other areas of functioning) need some degree of cognitive caregiving. As mild cognitive impairment progresses to more definite Alzheimer's disease, there is generally an increasing need for cognitive caregiving. Typical examples of cognitive caregiving include reminding the individual of appointments, medications, and other obligations.

Behavioral Caregiving

Behavioral caregiving can be defined as all of the time and energy (emotional and physical) spent on dealing with the various mood and behavioral symptoms and challenges of the person with Alzheimer's disease, which may include the following:

- Trying to calm the person with Alzheimer's who may seem too anxious to go to sleep
- Trying to cheer up someone who is very depressed over lost abilities
- Responding to concerns about "other people" in the house when no others are present
- Being the object of accusations of infidelity or other imagined transgressions
- Dealing with wandering
- A wide range of other symptoms and behaviors

It has been estimated that at least 90% of persons with Alzheimer's disease have one or more significant disturbances in their mood or conduct at some point during the course of the illness; at any given point in time, about half of all persons with the disease have at least one symptom of this type. Thus behavioral caregiving is a central component of the caregiving process for nearly everyone who has a loved one with the disease.

The different types of caregiving are separable only for the sake of discussion. In reality, caring for a loved one with Alzheimer's disease involves elements of passive, active, cognitive, and behavioral caregiving intermingled. Different types of caregiving are more or less stressful for different caregivers. As noted above, caring for bowel incontinence is one of the most stressful and disagreeable aspects of caregiving for nearly all caregivers. Other than that, however, most caregivers report that behavioral caregiving is the most stressful aspect of the disease. Significant behavioral symptoms can lead to early caregiver burnout and hastened nursing home placement. Dealing with behavioral symptoms is addressed separately in Chapter 7.

ADULT CHILDREN AS PRIMARY CAREGIVERS

When the spouse is also impaired with dementia or has significant physical illnesses, or when there is no living spouse, the task of primary caregiving falls to others. In our society, it is most commonly an adult daughter who assumes the responsibility of caring for her parent with dementia, if there is no spouse. If several adult daughters are nearby, the task will often fall to an unmarried daughter, if there is one. When no daughters are available, it is not uncommon for a son's wife (a daughter-in-law) to take on this task. Depending on the nature of the preexisting relationship between the daughter-in-law and the person with dementia, this can be a difficult situation. On the other hand, daughters-in-law usually don't have the long-standing complicated relationships that exist between adult children and their parents, so the caregiving relationship can be simpler, less burdened by unresolved issues. Less commonly, adult sons become primary caregivers, especially if there are no daughters nearby. Of course, depending on the particular family situation, the primary caregiver can be another relative or close friend.

For any adult child, becoming a primary or secondary caregiver for a parent with Alzheimer's inevitably involves a major reversal of roles; the parent who had been the caregiver for a significant portion of the child's life is now the care recipient, and vice versa. The child must now, in many ways, become the parent as the parent becomes the child. Adult children who have had positive and satisfying relationships with the parent—who feel good about the parenting given them by the one now afflicted with Alzheimer's—often develop a greater sense of closeness and a deep sense of satisfaction about being able to give back what was given to them earlier in life.

For adult children who have had more conflicted relationships, the situation is more difficult. Adult children who continue to feel controlled, unloved, overly criticized, or treated like a child by the parent will have a very difficult time stepping into the caregiver role. So will those who remain highly dependent on a parent whom they idealize, although their difficulties may be less apparent initially. Depending on the nature and severity of the underlying conflicts, some adult children will limit their involvement in caregiving. Others will participate, but often grudgingly and with little patience for the foibles of the person with Alzheimer's disease. These adult children tend to feel stressed and burdened by caregiving activities which those who have more healthy relationships find much less burdensome. One can sense that what they give, they give with a good deal of resentment.

The clinician working with these adult children needs to carefully explore the nature of the relationship prior to the parent becoming ill. For example, since becoming an adult, has there been significant genuine closeness, with little conflict? Or have conflicts from childhood and adolescence continued, in one form or another? Does the adult child feel genuine affection and respect for the afflicted parent? Does he or she enjoy their company, or remain in contact primarily out of a sense of guilt or obligation? Does the adult child feel loved and accepted, or does he or she continue to struggle to gain the approval of the parent? Many will initially indicate that their relationship has been strong; but more in-depth examination may reveal underlying, unresolved conflict.

While there is, of course, always a great amount of sadness whenever a loved one is diagnosed with Alzheimer's disease, it often appears that adult children with more conflicted relationships have more distress at that point than those whose parent-child relationship has been more mature and healthy. This is certainly not because those individuals feel any less love for their afflicted parent; but they do not have the added distress of unfinished emotional business contributing to their sadness.

For children (or other loved ones) who have conflicted relationships with the demented individual, although the diagnosis of Alzheimer's causes great sadness, it can also mark an important opportunity to try to heal the relationship before it is too late. This takes a great deal of work on the part of the family member and the clinician, and the clinician may need to repeatedly emphasize the importance of trying to bring the relationship to a more mature point, as there is usually a good deal of resistance on the part of the conflicted adult child. Yet in some ways, improving a relationship with a parent who has Alzheimer's disease may be easier than improving a troubled relationship with a parent who is cognitively intact. Perhaps this is because the situation forces the adult child to face the relationship more directly than when the parent is healthy. It may also be that children who have conflicted relationships with a parent often see that parent as extremely powerful or even intimidating, at least prior to the illness. Alzheimer's certainly renders the individual less powerful, more vulnerable, and often more approachable.

The situation may be more complicated in families where there has been overt abuse of the child by the person who now has dementia. Depending on the nature and severity of the abuse, adult children may have little desire to improve the relationship and may need to remain emotionally (and often physically) distant, for their own mental well-being. On the other hand, some abused adult children do use the opportunity of Alzheimer's to attempt to improve the relationship, or at least to feel that they can sufficiently overcome the past to become better care providers than the parent was to them. Or they may get involved only to ease the burden on the other parent or siblings. It is important to carefully explore this delicate situation with an abused adult child and not to assume that they are better off staying away, or that they should try to resolve the difficult relationship. The decision about whether to get involved in caregiving should only come from an in-depth discussion with the clinician regarding the relationship. In most cases, unless the abuse was very severe, adult childen will choose to get involved and will feel less guilty in the long run if they do. However, the discussion and decision making about this can be of lasting value to adult children, whether or not they decide to get involved.

When there are several adult children, they may be able to work cooperatively to care for a parent with Alzheimer's, and the strengths of sibling bonds can be quite impressive. However, just as some parent-child relationships remain troubled into adulthood, there are dysfunctional sibling relationships as well. When this is the case, adult siblings may have little contact with each other until a parent is in need of care, but then the unresolved conflicts between siblings can surge to the surface. In advising an adult child with troubled sibling relationships, it is important for clinicians to explore the history of these relationships in depth, just as they do with dysfunctional parent-child relationships. It is rarely the case that siblings who have gotten along well throughout life will begin to have difficulties purely as a result of the need to pro-

vide care for a parent with Alzheimer's. Most of the time, exploring those relationships in depth reveals long-standing and
unresolved sibling rivalries and resentments.

Being forced to work together to care for an ailing parent may
or may not significantly improve the sibling relationship, but it is
certainly important to minimize the impact of the sibling tension
on the person with Alzheimer's disease. Even significantly demented parents can sense difficulties between their children and
can become quite upset by it. Often the difficulties between siblings manifest in complaints from one sibling that one or more of
the other siblings do not help sufficiently (or at all) with the caregiving tasks. It is not uncommon that when several siblings live
near the person with Alzheimer's disease, there is significant imbalance in how much caregiving each does. As noted above, when
there is one unmarried sibling, particularly a female, most of the
tasks seem to fall to her. It is common for this person to feel deeply
angry and resentful toward her siblings. She may feel that they
take advantage of her as the one who does not have a spouse and
her own children to care for. This may be an accurate picture of
what actually occurs. On a deeper level, the unmarried sibling
may feel that her brothers and sisters have been dealt a better
hand in life, with spouses and children, and she is left, like Cin-
derella, to do the dirty work. It is important to bring these feelings
to the surface and to try to help establish a fairer balance of caregiving duties among the available siblings. When there are multiple siblings, each one should have at least one caregiving task. For
one sibling, that might be handing the finances; another may plow
the snow in winter, mow the lawn in summer, and do minor house
maintenance; another sibling may be the one who gives her afflicted mother a weekly shampoo and manicure. Another sibling's
task may be to assist financially, if he or she is in a position to do so
but is not able (or willing) to do much hands-on care. Dividing up
tasks like this is critical so that the family as whole can be involved
in caregiving in one way or another. This approach will go a long
way to lessen (although perhaps not eliminate) the resentment felt
by the sibling who has been designated as the primary caregiver.

What about adult children who live a considerable distance

from the parent with Alzheimer's disease? When siblings live too far away to participate regularly in care, their job may be to come home every so often to stay with the person with Alzheimer's disease so that the primary sibling (or spouse) may have some respite. It is important to realize that these family members who are not regularly involved in providing supervision or care can nevertheless be deeply affected by the illness. Predominant emotions in those who live far from an impaired loved one are sadness, of course, and guilt that by living so far away they are not able to be involved (or are spared of being involved) in the day-to-day care of their family member. There is often a sense of frustration about being able to do so little from such a distance, and there may be anger or resentment toward those who are closer at hand and are managing the situation in ways that the distant relative feels are incorrect. Often those at a distance have a very different view of the status and needs of the person with Alzheimer's. These long-distance family members can greatly benefit from seeing a clinician to help them cope with the stresses of their position.

If a family member develops Alzheimer's, it can be an important opportunity to attempt to improve dysfunctional relationships between family members. When that is possible, it is enormously gratifying for all. At other times, family tensions that were ignored prior to the illness only worsen when someone develops Alzheimer's and remain intense despite all efforts to improve the situation. At these times, earlier placement in a long-term care facility may actually be best for the individual with Alzheimer's, to remove him or her from the toxic environment caused by family discord. Fortunately, this is relatively uncommon.

CHAPTER 2

Memory Loss and Dementia: Understanding the Basics

Alzheimer's disease is the most common cause of serious memory loss in older people, but it is certainly not the only cause of cognitive decline. It is important to be certain that appropriate consideration has been given to a number of other conditions, and not assume that everyone who is forgetful is suffering from Alzheimer's disease.

One of the interesting but challenging issues that clinicians and researchers face today is that there are no definite diagnostic markers for Alzheimer's disease or, for that matter, for most other types of dementia or other cognitive impairment. The changes in memory that occur as a result of aging, the changes of so-called mild cognitive impairment (MCI, see below), and the changes of Alzheimer's disease all exist on a continuum with no firm lines of demarcation. We may be getting close to having a biomarker for Alzheimer's disease, but, at present, the diagnosis of this condition is based on clinical judgment. That is to say, the clinician gathers the history from the patient and, ideally, the family; performs a thorough mental status examination including cognitive examination; and reviews laboratory findings, neuroimaging studies, and any other relevant information that is available. Using all of these data (which may be collected all at once or over a period of time), the clinician develops a diagnostic impression. When the diagnostic impression is Alzheimer's disease, clinicians who are experienced in evaluating these individuals (e.g., doctors who work in memory clinics or other specialty settings) have about a 90% accuracy rate, based on research (Kosunen, 1996) that has followed patients to autopsy. However, when the person has more atypical symptoms, or when the evaluation is not done by a specialist, the percentage of accurate diagnosis is probably lower.

There is even greater ambiguity when the issue is whether or not the person has MCI, some other cause of memory loss, or simply the normal changes in memory and thinking that are seen in aging. Here, the diagnostic criteria are more vague; the situation can change in either direction over time, and clinicians will have more trouble agreeing on what is wrong, if anything.

Despite these difficulties, it is quite important for clinicians to be as precise as possible about the causes of someone's cognitive difficulties. It is important not to diagnose Alzheimer's disease or other dementia when the problem is less serious and possibly more reversible; but it is equally important to make a positive diagnosis of Alzheimer's when it is present, so that the patient and family can become aware of the nature of the problem and plan around it, and so that treatment can begin. And it is certainly crucial to know if cognitive difficulties are due to a potentially treatable medical or psychological condition, or to medications that may have been prescribed for another illness.

COGNITIVE CHANGES ASSOCIATED WITH AGING

Perhaps the most common cognitive change is the difficulty people have remembering names as they age. Actually, the declining ability to remember names begins in midlife but becomes more noticeable by age 60 or sometimes even earlier. Typically, we will have no trouble recognizing people we know; we will be able to describe where they live, how many children they have, what they do for a living, and perhaps even more trivial details about their lives—everything, in short, but a name. Eventually, the name may come, but not always. This can be enormously frustrating, even embarrassing, but when it is not severe (e.g., if not every name is forgotten) and if it is not accompanied by other cognitive changes, it is most likely just a sign of aging.

Another change that is extremely common with age is a slight decline in immediate recall, one manifestation of which is the common but frustrating phenomenon of going from one room of the house to another to get something, and forgetting what was being sought once arriving there. Another change that is nearly ubiquitous is a decline in the ability to multitask. Young adults are able to talk on a cell phone, check and answer e-mail, keep an eye on a ballgame on television, and read an article in a magazine or chapter in a textbook—all at the same time (just ask the parent of any teenager about this). As we age, it gets more and more difficult and eventually impossible to do even two of these tasks at the same time. We are no longer able to split our attention in several different directions, but need to maintain our focus on just one thing at a time. If we try to do more than one of these tasks at once, the accuracy of each task attempted diminishes significantly.

POTENTIALLY REVERSIBLE CAUSES OF COGNITIVE IMPAIRMENT

Emotional, Psychological, and Physical Stressors That Can Affect Memory

Just as teens and young adults can multitask, while seniors cannot, older individuals, overall, tend to have less ability to maintain their cognitive abilities when stressed by various factors, compared to their younger counterparts. This means that when a younger individual is weighed down by depression, anxiety, or some other type of emotional stress, or a mild physical illness such as an upper respiratory infection or bladder infection, he or she is generally able to function at or close to normal cognitively, unless the physical or emotional stress is quite severe. Older individuals, on the other hand, and particularly those who may have even a very mild degree of cognitive impairment, are much more affected by any stressor, mental or physical: depression, anxiety, insomnia, or other emotional stress; a mild (or, certainly, severe) physical illness, or certain medications, to mention the most common examples. Under these circumstances, the older individual may show a significant decline in memory, speed of thinking, concentration ability, word finding, and other cognitive abilities. Older persons often lack the ability to tolerate a challenge to their system without having it impact their thinking.

Generally, the stresses mentioned above are transient; for example, an upper respiratory infection is a self-limited event. While older people may show significant cognitive difficulties during such an illness, it is expected that they will return to baseline once they are fully well, although there can be some delay. In the case of more serious or lasting illnesses, the impact on cognition can be more marked, and may not be reversible, depending on the illness. For example, many patients who undergo life-saving open-heart surgery or cancer chemotherapy have lingering and often permanent cognitive effects from these treatments.

However, emotional stressors may be harder to identify and can persist for a long time, especially if not recognized. When an older individual is assessed for complaints about memory, it is critical to determine if he or she is suffering from depression, anxiety, significant stress from a difficult psychosocial situation, insomnia, or unusual emotional challenge.

Alcohol and Other Substances

Among the elderly, the most commonly abused substances are alcohol and prescription medications. While there is some evidence that one or two standard servings of alcohol per day may be beneficial to general health, or at least not harmful, higher amounts of daily alcohol intake are definitely associated with an increased risk of dementia. And for anyone with even mild degrees of cognitive impairment, any amount of alcohol consumption can at least temporarily worsen cognition. It is not known if modest alcohol intake is harmful for the person who already has cognitive impairment, but the immediate effects of one or two drinks on memory and thinking can be quite marked. It can be a challenge to get anyone to stop drinking, particularly if a degree of substance dependence is present, but it may be important for the clinician to address this with the family member who is concerned about the memory function of a loved one. Many older individuals (even more so than younger adults) are reluctant to admit the amount of alcohol they consume, and they may not answer alcohol screening questions in a way that accurately describes their usual alcohol consumption patterns. Often a family member will report the amount of alcohol consumed as significantly greater than the patient will acknowledge. While it is certainly possible that family members may exaggerate, their report is often more accurate overall than that of the person with cognitive problems. This may be true because of a conscious reluctance on the part of the individual to admit the degree of use, as well as more classic denial. Of course the individual may also be unable to correctly remember the amount being consumed. The clinician should advise the family not to get into a debate with their loved one about how much he or she is drinking or about addiction, but to simply reinforce that any alcohol consumption in someone with memory problems has the potential to make the situation worse.

Other drugs of abuse are less commonly used by this population (other than prescription medications), but if other substance abuse is present in someone who has cognitive issues, that needs to be addressed urgently, as it is likely a major contributor to the cognitive decline. The clinician can perhaps be helpful in making a referral to a substance abuse specialist. Before any definitive diagnosis of an underlying cognitive illness can be made, it is essential that the substance abuse issues are addressed.

Medications That Can Affect Thinking and Memory

When there is a concern about memory impairment, all prescription and nonprescription medications the individual is currently taking should be thoroughly reviewed. It is quite common for older people to take numerous medications, a great many of which can affect memory and thinking. This includes most of the medications used for anxiety or insomnia, and many for depression. As noted above, the most commonly abused substances among the elderly (after alcohol) are prescription medications, usually hypnotics, pain medications, or benzodiazepines (e.g., lorazepam, alprazolam) given for anxiety.

In addition, a great many compounds that are used to treat conditions unrelated to the brain or central nervous system can nevertheless have a significant adverse impact on the neurotransmitter acetylcholine. This can be useful for various medical conditions, but these compounds can also lessen cholinergic transmission in the brain, which can lead to impairment in short-term memory. Medications that have so-called anticholinergic properties are used for overactive bladder or gastrointestinal reflux, hypertension, Parkinson's disease, allergies, and breathing disorders, to name just a few. It has been estimated that half of all seniors take at least one anticholinergic medication. The following are some of the most commonly used anticholinergic medications:

Antidepressants
- Amoxapine
- Amitriptyline
- Clomipramine
- Desipramine
- Doxepin
- Imipramine
- Nortriptyline
- Protriptyline
- Paroxetine

Antihistamines
- Chlorpheniramine
- Cyproheptadine
- Diphenhydramine
- Hydroxyzine

Antipsychotics
- Chlorpromazine
- Clozapine
- Olanzapine
- Thioridazine

Cardiovascular medications
- Furosemide
- Digoxin
- Nifedipine
- Disopyramide

Gastrointestinal medications
- Antidiarrheal
  ◦ Diphenoxylate
  ◦ Atropine
- Antispasmodic
  ◦ Belladonna
  ◦ Clidinium
  ◦ Chlordiazepoxide
  ◦ Dicyclomine
  ◦ Hyoscyamine
  ◦ Propantheline
  ◦ Cimetidine
  ◦ Ranitidine
- Medications for nausea
  ◦ Prochlorperazine
  ◦ Promethazine

Medications for vertigo
- Meclizine
- Scopolamine

Muscle relaxants
- Cyclobenzaprine
- Dantrolene
- Orphenadrine

Medications for Parkinson's symptoms
- Amantadine
- Benztropine
- Biperiden
- Trihexyphenidyl

Medications for urinary incontinence and overactive bladder
- Oxybutynin
- Propantheline

- Solifenacin
- Tolterodine
- Trospium

At times, it can be difficult to tell whether the disease itself or the medication being used to treat it is the cause of cognitive worsening. A prime example of this is levodopa/carbidopa, a medication that is absolutely vital for many persons with Parkinson's disease to maintain mobility and to decrease the other debilitating motor symptoms of the illness. Both Parkinson's disease and levodopa/carbidopa can cause cognitive confusion and other mental symptoms, and it can be difficult to tell which is the real culprit.

Even over-the-counter medications, which many individuals (erroneously) feel are completely safe because they do not require a prescription, can cause significant cognitive effects. Most prominent among these is diphenhydramine, a common allergy and cold remedy that is also used as a sleep aid. It is the chief ingredient of many over-the-counter sleeping medications, sometimes mixed with acetaminophen or other agents. Diphenhydramine is significantly anticholinergic and should be avoided by people who have cognitive difficulties.

Delirium

An important and usually reversible cause of cognitive impairment is a medical condition called delirium. Delirium is sometimes called *metabolic encephalopathy, acute brain failure*, or a variety of other terms. Delirium is generally a reaction to a single physical stressor or a combination of stressors in a vulnerable individual. For example, a high fever or an infection in the blood can cause delirium. In older individuals, delirium can be caused by factors such as a urinary tract infection, anesthesia, medications (in addition to the anticholinergic effects described above), withdrawal from alcohol or other addictive substances, or a wide variety of other conditions. Common symptoms of delirium include a sudden change in mental status characterized by inattention, confusion, changes in levels of alertness, and sometimes hallucinations.

Symptoms can be present at one point in time but will vary greatly and may be completely absent minutes or hours later, only to return again. The recognition and treatment of delirium is considered a medical emergency, because persons who are delirious can be quite dangerous to themselves, intentionally or inadvertently. Also, the longer a state of delirium continues, the greater the chance that the victim may suffer permanent cognitive damage. When delirium is discovered and treated promptly, the florid symptoms go away completely, restoring individuals to their former state.

The treatment of delirium involves determining the underlying cause and reversing it when possible. For example, if the delirium is due to an infection, appropriate antibiotic therapy needs to be given. If the cause is a toxic reaction to a medication, the medication needs to be identified and stopped, if at all possible. If the cause is alcohol or drug withdrawal, certain benzodiazepines are usually given to lessen or eliminate the symptoms. Delirium not due to alcohol or drug withdrawal may also need treatment with antipsychotic medications, such as haloperidol or quetiapine, if the delirious individual is quite agitated or hallucinating.

Delirium is common in the elderly, and it is most common in individuals who have an underlying dementia. When that is the case, it can at times be difficult to tease out the symptoms that are due to delirium from the underlying symptoms of dementia, but generally the demented individual who becomes delirious has a sudden worsening of confusion, a greater degree of inattentiveness than before, and wide fluctuations in mental status over the course of brief periods of time. Sudden changes in mental status are not usually seen in dementia unless there is also an underlying delirium.

Frequently, there is no single factor causing delirium, but a variety of stressors (e.g., high fever, systemic infection, high doses of pain medications, and a baseline of cognitive impairment) that can reach a tipping point and produce delirium. When that is the case, it may be more difficult (but no less important) to identify the contributing factors and address each of them as effectively as possible.

MILD COGNITIVE IMPAIRMENT

If cognitive ability is viewed as existing on a continuum, with completely normal thinking at one end and severe Alzheimer's disease on the other, MCI falls somewhere in between. Mild cognitive impairment is a term that describes changes in memory that clearly go beyond those of normal aging, but without significant impairments in function, which is necessary for a diagnosis of Alzheimer's disease. Some researchers have found that a very high percentage of cases of MCI progress to Alzheimer's disease, while others have found a much lower rate of conversion, with some persons with MCI improving back to normal cognition. What is clear is that there are indeed people who fall somewhere between the normal cognitive changes associated with aging, on the one hand, and Alzheimer's disease on the other. Some of these individuals are without doubt on the way to Alzheimer's disease, but at present there is no definitive way to determine which patients with MCI will progress to Alzheimer's disease, and which will not. MCI may be a rather heterogeneous condition, with a variety of etiologies and outcomes.

In addition to the uncertain prognosis for people with MCI, there is no approved treatment for this condition. Most studies of treatment for MCI have not found the antidementia medications to have lasting benefit.

While there are clear research criteria for MCI, based on neuropsychological testing differences from normals of the same age and education level, in practice, it may be quite difficult for a clinician, following a clinical interview or even a brief office cognitive test, to determine whether or not someone has MCI. An experienced clinician may develop a strong suspicion based on being able to informally compare the person's cognitive abilities to many others seen; while this may be an educated guess, it is still a guess.

DEMENTIA

On the spectrum of cognitive impairment discussed above, dementia is on the far end, more severe than MCI, and well beyond the typical cognitive changes of aging. According to the American Psychiatric Association's *Diagnostic and Statistical Manual of Mental Disorders* (4th ed.; 1994), a diagnosis of dementia requires impairment in memory and at least one other cognitive domain, sufficient to cause significant impairment in daily functioning. In addition, the symptoms must represent a significant change from the previous level of functioning, and cannot be due to delirium or another disorder.

The most common types of dementia are as follows:

- Mixed dementia
- Vascular dementia
- Dementia with Lewy bodies
- Dementia due to Parkinson's disease
- Frontotemporal dementia
- Alzheimer's disease

In addition to these more common causes of dementia, a number of other illnesses can also cause dementia, including Huntington's disease, Creutzfelt-Jakob disease, normal-pressure hydrocephalus, brain tumors, severe head trauma, untreated metabolic conditions such as hypothyroidism, hypoxic brain injury, multiple sclerosis, chronic alcoholism, and HIV/AIDS, to name just a few. While it is very important for clinicians to try to be precise about the exact diagnosis of a dementing illness, that is sometimes not possible with our current knowledge and technology. The specific signs and symptoms of Alzheimer's disease, risk factors for the disease, and the course of illness are all discussed in more detail below.

Mixed Dementia and Vascular Dementia

It used to be thought that dementia caused by vascular disease (i.e., vascular dementia) was the second most common form of dementia, after Alzheimer's disease, and that belief continues to be widespread. In fact, studies based on brain autopsies of persons with dementia have found that pure vascular dementia is less common than previously thought, accounting for a relatively small percentage of cases. These are patients whose brains show single or more frequently multiple areas of vascular disease (small or large brain infarcts), but they do not have the classic pathology of Alzheimer's disease (plaques and tangles) or of other conditions (e.g., Lewy bodies in Lewy body dementia and Parkinson's dementia). Much more common are cases where vascular disease and pathologic features of Alzheimer's disease are mixed together. Such cases are called *mixed dementia*. Clinically (i.e., before death), the diagnosis of mixed dementia is made when there is evidence of vascular disease of the brain, either by history or with neuroimaging, yet also a classic history of Alzheimer's disease or a family history of Alzheimer's disease. In practice, it is usually not possible to say whether a person who has clinical evidence for vascular disease of the brain and also has clinical signs of dementia has vascular disease alone, or (more commonly) Alzheimer's pathology as well. Based on statistics alone, the latter is much more likely. Individuals who have been normal cognitively, and then have a significant stroke that leads to cognitive impairment but then no further strokes and no further cognitive decline for a considerable period of time may have pure vascular dementia. One day, hopefully soon, we will have tests that permit us to make these differential diagnostic decisions with great accuracy. For now, we must rely on clinical judgment, which is never 100% accurate.

Does it matter? Why would it be important to know the exact nature of the patient's dementia, if that were possible? One reason it matters is because Alzheimer's disease has a typical course of progressive cognitive decline, even with current treatments, while vascular dementia may not be progressive if no further vascular events occur. Also, Alzheimer's disease more commonly runs in families, so the children of the victim will be more likely to develop Alzheimer's if a parent has it. Finally, the medications currently available for Alzheimer's disease have been tested and proven effective in that condition, but less is known about their effectiveness in pure vascular dementia.

When a patient presents with cognitive decline suggestive of dementia, with some evidence of vascular disease on brain imaging, but has a typical history of progressive and gradual cognitive decline, the clinician should assume that Alzheimer's disease pathology is present and treat the patient accordingly. Not infrequently, clinicians erroneously assume that a person with, for example, hypertension or diabetes (risk factors for vascular disease) and dementia has vascular dementia. In fact, most of the risk factors for vascular disease are also risk factors for Alzheimer's disease, and most of those patients will turn out to have Alzheimer's disease, whether or not there is also vascular disease of the brain.

Lewy Body Dementia

After Alzheimer's disease, and mixed dementia, Lewy body dementia may be the most common cause of dementia. Lewy body dementia (also called diffuse Lewy body disease, dementia with Lewy bodies, or simply DLB) appears clinically to be a mixture of Alzheimer's disease and Parkinson's disease. While the specific symptoms in a person with DLB do vary, a core feature of Lewy body dementia is markedly fluctuating levels of cognition with great variations in attention and alertness from day to day or even hour to hour. In addition, up to 75% of persons with DLB have visual hallucinations. And they have at least some of the motor features of Parkinson's disease: an expressionless face, stooped posture, shuffling gait, a resting tremor, or a tendency to fall.

From the caregiver's standpoint, DLB can be especially challenging for several reasons: The marked fluctuations from relative lucidity to significant confusion can be difficult to understand or manage, particularly if the caregiver has not been informed that this is a common feature of the disease. Also, the frequent presence of hallucinations, as well as other behavioral disturbances, can be particularly challenging. Persons with DLB do poorly with antipsychotic medications, which should be avoided, so other means must be found to deal with hallucinations and other psychotic features when they occur. Finally, as the disease progresses, the increasing physical impairment due to Parkinsonism requires a considerable and increasing degree of physical care, more than most caregivers are able to provide without outside assistance.

People with Lewy body dementia often respond to antidementia medications, although such medications do not help the physical (parkinsonian) symptoms. Antiparkinson medications such as levodopa/carbidopa are variably helpful for the motor symptoms of DLB but do not help the cognitive symptoms.

Parkinson's Dementia

Parkinson's disease occurs about one tenth as frequently as Alzheimer's disease, but that still makes it a common illness. Currently, about 500,000 persons in the United States suffer from Parkinson's disease. Usually, dementia does not occur until Parkinson's disease has been present for at least 1 to 2 years. Overall, about 30–40% of persons with Parkinson's disease will develop dementia, increasing with the duration of the illness to as much as 75% of long-standing Parkinson's disease patients (Ceravolo et al., 2010; Chaudhuri et al., 2006).

The onset of dementia relative to the onset of motor symptoms helps differentiate Parkinson's dementia from Lewy body dementia. Patients with Parkinson's disease must have had motor symptoms for at least 1 year prior to the onset of cognitive symptoms, but in Lewy body disease, the cognitive symptoms and motor symptoms begin about the same time. While this seems clear on paper, in practice it can sometimes be difficult to differentiate the two conditions.

Only one medication is currently approved by the FDA for the treatment of dementia associated with Parkinson's disease—rivastigmine. While it can be helpful in lessening or temporarily stabilizing the cognitive symptoms, it certainly does not cure them, and the disease will continue to progress, unfortunately. Medications used to treat the motor symptoms of Parkinson's disease (e.g., levodopa/carbidopa, benztropine, and the like) will frequently worsen the cognitive symptoms of the disease, so careful medical management is needed.

Frontotemporal Dementia

Frontotemporal dementia (FTD) stands somewhat apart from the other dementias. The age of onset tends to be somewhat younger, on average, than the other dementias; and, notably, patients may have relatively preserved memory compared to other functions, at least early in the disease. Persons with FTD tend to fall into two categories: those with prominent apathy, and those with disinhibited behaviors. Both groups have significant problems with executive function: Patients have significant difficulty performing tasks that require complex planning or the sequencing of activities. Eventually, memory and language become very impaired, and these individuals almost always need full-time, usually institutional, care later in the disease. Unfortunately, there are no effective treatments for FTD. About 5–10% of all cases of dementia are frontotemporal. Although frontotemporal dementia was formerly considered a single disease, more recently several types have been identified, the most common of which is Pick's disease. A detailed discussion of the various types of FTD is beyond the scope of this book.

Alzheimer's Disease

Alzheimer's disease is the most common form of dementia, by far, accounting for well over half of all cases (Querfurth et al., 2010). It is a type of dementia, not a totally different condition, as many people seem to believe. All people with Alzheimer's disease have dementia; but not all people with dementia have Alzheimer's disease. That may change in the future, if and when it becomes possible to definitively diagnose Alzheimer's disease (via blood or spinal fluid test, neuroimaging, or other methods) before there are any clinical signs of illness. If that occurs, it may be possible to determine that someone has Alzheimer's disease before any signs of dementia are present. But for now, the diagnosis of Alzheimer's disease requires that the individual meet criteria for dementia (described above). In addition, the symptoms cannot be caused by any other illness, and the course of illness is described as having an insidious onset and progressive cognitive decline. These features are often the most helpful in being able to determine that an individual's illness is likely Alzheimer's disease, rather than another form of dementia.

RISK FACTORS FOR ALZHEIMER'S DISEASE

Age

Age is the greatest risk factor, by far, for Alzheimer's disease. While only about 2% of the population at age 65 has Alzheimer's disease, the incidence of the disease doubles every 5 years, so that by age 85, about 40% of those still living meet criteria for Alzheimer's disease. Since females generally live longer than males, there are more women living with Alzheimer's disease than men.

Genetic Factors

In addition to age, genetics play an important role in determining one's risk for the disease. While it is likely that many genes play some role in the development of Alzheimer's, only one has been shown to confer significant risk—the apolipoprotein E gene, found on chromosome 21. The gene has three different alleles: E2, E3, and E4.

Each individual has one chromosome from each parent. The most common genetic pattern is E3/E3; that is, the individual has inherited an E3 from each parent. This is said to be the neutral condition. However, if someone inherits one E4, the risk of developing Alzheimer's increases significantly. How E4 exerts this effect is not clear. Although 40–65% of Alzheimer's patients have at least one copy of the E4 allele, at least a third of patients do not have any APO E4; and some individuals with two APO E4s never develop the disease. While 25–30% of the population carries an APO E4 allele, 40% of those with Alzheimer's disease have at least one E4. If an individual inherits an E4 from each parent, the risk of developing Alzheimer's disease is very much greater than in those with no E4, and the onset of symptoms tends to be earlier. If, on the other hand, one inherits an E2, it lowers the risk of developing Alzheimer's. Having one E4 and one E2 neutralizes the risk, and these individuals have the same risk of developing the disease as those who have two E3s. Apparently, having two E2s is not compatible with life, for reasons which are unclear.

While APO E is clearly important, this gene is merely a risk factor for Alzheimer's, and not an inevitable cause of the disease. For this reason, it is not recommended that individuals be tested for this genotype. Finding that one has no E4 allele could provide false reassurance, while having one or two E4s could lead to considerable distress, when at present there is nothing that can be done to effectively prevent the disease from developing. Nevertheless, some individuals strongly desire to learn their APO E status, particularly when they have a parent and other relatives with the disease. It would be important for the clinician to discuss the pros and cons of obtaining this test before any decision is made, and a referral to a genetic counselor may be worthwhile.

Having a parent or a sibling (i.e., a first-degree relative) with Alzheimer's statistically increases the risk of developing the disease by a factor of two to three. Having two parents with the disease is associated with an even greater risk to each offspring. These individuals—particularly those with two parents who have the disease—need to be followed closely over time, and even without the benefit of genetic tests should be encouraged to do whatever they can to lower the risk of getting the disease, or delay its onset (see next section).

Other Risk Factors for Alzheimer's Disease

In addition to age and genetics, a number of other factors have been associated with an increased risk of developing the disease. These are modifiable risk factors, unlike age and genetic status. That is, the individual may be able to lower the risk of developing Alzheimer's by following some specific approaches. Firm cause-and-effect relationships have not been established for these factors but merely statistical associations. In some cases, it would seem obvious that the factor causes or contributes to cognitive worsening. In other situations, there may be a third factor that influences both the factor being considered and the prevalence of the disease. Determining the exact causal relationship for these matters would be nearly impossible scientifically. Nevertheless, in the absence of absolute preventive measures or dramatically effective treatments, is seems valuable to pursue some of these strategies. In addition to possibly lowering the risk of developing Alzheimer's disease, in most cases these measures are good for one's health and well-being generally. And these interventions are generally very safe.

Cardiovascular Factors

It has been determined over the last decade that factors which increase the risk of heart disease also increase the risk of Alzheimer's disease. Importantly, interventions that lessen the risk of heart disease also lower the risk of Alzheimer's. Thus it is known that high blood pressure, obesity, lack of physical exercise, high cholesterol, and diabetes—all risk factors for heart disease—are also independent risk factors for Alzheimer's disease. Similarly, interventions designed to improve these conditions—for example, lowering blood pressure with diet, following a regular exercise regimen, losing weight if necessary, or antihypertensive medications—will decrease the risk of Alzheimer's disease. While the exact mechanism is not known, it is thought that it has to do with preserving a healthy vascular system.

Similarly, a diet that is low in fat and cholesterol and moderate in caloric intake not only lowers the risk of heart disease but may also decrease the risk of Alzheimer's. There is some evidence, as well, that consuming significant amounts of fruits and vegetables with folates and antioxidants may also contribute to both heart health and brain health. Thus it is commonly said that what's good for the heart is good for the brain.

Lifestyle Risk Factors

Lifestyle factors play a role as well. Excessive consumption of alcohol or cigarette smoking increases the risk of dementia from a variety of causes, including Alzheimer's disease. It has been known for some time that significant head injury, particularly one associated with prolonged loss of consciousness, at any time in life brings higher risks, for reasons that are not fully clear. Education and general intellectual enrichment throughout life may help build "cognitive reserve" so that later in life, if one begins to develop the brain-damaging pathology of Alzheimer's disease, there is literally more reserve—possibly more synapses or more neurons—to protect against developing cognitive symptoms in the face of the loss of brain neurons with the disease. This is why those with more education still get the disease but may develop the clinical picture later, and then progress somewhat more rapidly, compressing the time of disability somewhat compared to those with less education and presumably less cognitive reserve.

Interesting studies have noted that individuals who have enhanced human connections throughout life—not only more connections with others, but more satisfying ones—may have a lower risk of developing Alzheimer's disease. And individuals who keep themselves mentally active in late life may be less inclined to develop the disease. Here it is very difficult to determine cause and effect; it may simply be that persons who are able to remain cognitively engaged in late life are not likely to get Alzheimer's in the first place, whereas those who are less active mentally may be that way because there are very subtle changes in their cognitive functions—precursors of Alzheimer's—that make them disinclined to pursue intellectual pursuits in the first place.

BRAIN PATHOLOGY IN ALZHEIMER'S DISEASE

Alois Alzheimer, a German neuropathologist and psychiatrist, first described the brain pathology of his patient, Auguste Deter, about 100 years ago. Auguste suffered from what would now be called early-onset Alzheimer's disease. The condition was named after Dr. Alzheimer sometime after his death, by his colleague, Dr. Emil Kraepelin. Originally, the term *Alzheimer's disease* applied only to those individuals who, like Auguste Deter, developed the disease before age 65. The much more common later-onset dementia was referred to simply as senile (i.e., over 65) dementia. Much later, it was recognized that the two diseases are identical, except for the age of onset, and so the later-onset dementia also was identified as late-onset Alzheimer's disease while the original illness in younger persons was called presenile or early-onset dementia. Because it was only much later that the more common late-onset version was also called Alzheimer's disease, there are

still some practitioners who think of Alzheimer's disease as a relatively rare condition.

In any case, after her death, Dr. Alzheimer performed an autopsy on the brain of Auguste Deter and was able to stain thin
slices of brain tissue so that the pathology of the disease would be
visible under the microscope. Dr. Alzheimer first identified the
"senile plaques and neurofibrillary tangles" that are known to this
day as the hallmark of the pathology of this condition. Amyloid
plaques are dense accumulations of amyloid precursor protein,
bound together and sitting in the connective tissue outside of the
brain neurons. Neurofibrillary tangles, on the other hand, are
characteristic accumulations of abnormal tau protein that gather
inside the nerve cell, disrupting transportation of nutrients and
other materials through the axons of the cell.

Because there is no biomarker or other test that can be done
during life to confirm the diagnosis of Alzheimer's disease, it is
only after death, on pathological examination of the patient's brain
tissue, that a firm diagnosis can be made. This is done by counting
the numbers of plaques and tangles found in one so-called high-
power field—the area that can be seen though the microscope
when one looks with a large degree of magnification. If there are
sufficient numbers of plaques and tangles, the diagnosis of Alzheimer's disease is made.

How plaques and tangles form and how they cause damage to
the brain in ways that ultimately lead to Alzheimer's disease is
beyond the scope of this book. In addition, numerous other pathologic processes have been identified in the brains of persons with
the disease. Unfortunately, although much is known about the pathology associated with the disease, it is still not known what
causes Alzheimer's disease—what sets off the cascade of events
that ultimately leads to brain cell death and the loss of memory,
functioning, and other domains that are known as Alzheimer's disease. Only when there is a clearer idea of why this happens in the
first place will effective treatments be developed or, better yet, a
method of preventing it from developing in the first place. It would
appear that the goal of preventing Alzheimer's disease is still some
distance away, unfortunately.

COGNITIVE, FUNCTIONAL, AND BEHAVIORAL SYMPTOMS OF ALZHEIMER'S DISEASE

It is said that "when you've seen one person with Alzheimer's disease, you've only seen one person with Alzheimer's disease." Just as no two people without Alzheimer's are alike in many respects, no two people with Alzheimer's disease are alike, even though there are characteristic symptoms and features of the disease.

Alzheimer's specialists often refer to the ABCs of Alzheimer's, referring to the areas of impairment that typically occur in the disease: activities, behavior, and cognition. To this alphabet, one can add a D, as well—the drain on the caregiver and family. Thinking about the ABCDs of Alzheimer's emphasizes that it is really impossible to consider the impairments of Alzheimer's disease without considering their impact on the caregiver and family as well; this is indeed a family illness. The paragraphs that follow describe the typical activities, behavior, and cognitive impairments; the remainder of this book addresses D, the impact of the disease on the caregiver and family, and vice versa.

A Is for Activities

Activities refers to the so-called instrumental activities of daily living (IADLs) and the basic activities of daily living (ADLs). Instrumental activities are higher-level functions, requiring a greater degree of cognitive acuity, which tend to become impaired earlier in the disease process. IADLs include such things as balancing a checkbook, paying bills, cooking, shopping, using electronics (microwave, cell phone, ATM, and the like), and driving. Of course, these don't decline all at once. Nor is it the case that one day a person is capable of performing a task and the next day is completely unable to do so. IADLs, like everything else in Alzheimer's disease, decline gradually, although the impairment in a particular activity—driving, for example—may reach a tipping point that alerts others to the problem. The tipping point might be an accident or getting lost. While behaviors are declining, the individual is often unaware of it and may be quite resistant to the notion that something is wrong. But when the tipping point is reached—an accident or getting lost while driving, or having the power turned off because of neglecting to pay the electric bill, for example—the individual is no longer able to hide his difficulties, and the family may become aware, for the first time, that there are functional problems, along with memory issues.

Driving is one of the more critical IADLs, as it involves critical issues of personal autonomy and independence, personal safety, and the safety of others. Driving is discussed in more detail in Chapter 6.

Basic ADLs include dressing, feeding oneself, using the toilet, bathing and general hygiene, and walking. Usually these activities become impaired later in the disease process, after the IADLs are already significantly compromised. Dressing is frequently the first ADL to become impaired. Individuals with early to moderate Alzheimer's disease may begin to have difficulties with choosing correct clothing and may put on summer shorts when it is snowing, or put two or three shirts on, or put a bra on outside the shirt. If clothing is laid out, they may be able to dress correctly or may need some cueing (e.g., "Put on your socks before you put on your shoes," or "Let me help you with those pants" which are going on backwards). As the disease progresses, they may need assistance with tying shoes or buttoning buttons. Later, it may become necessary to dress them completely.

Problems with eating usually begin with the individual becoming very messy at the table, no longer recognizing the correct utensil for a particular food (e.g., attempting to eat soup with a fork), spitting food out onto the plate or the floor, and using fingers to eat items that are not finger food (e.g., mashed potatoes).

Difficulty with toileting is, of course, a challenging issue for caregivers to handle. Males, in particular, may urinate in inappropriate locations, such as the garbage pail, the sink, a potted plant, or simply on the floor, because the toilet is no longer recognized or remembered. Incontinence often begins at night, in bed for both sexes, although that can be variable. Urinary continence tends to be lost before bowel continence, but accidents may occur intermittently prior to losing continence entirely. Once patients lose bowel continence entirely, caregivers frequently feel they can no longer care for the individual at home; bowel incontinence is one of the chief precipitants of nursing home placement, along with behavioral problems (see next section).

Usually, the final ADL to become impaired (unless there are other physical reasons to have difficulties earlier) is the ability to walk. Persons in the later stages of dementia may literally become too cognitively impaired to know how to put one foot safely in front of the other. They suffer frequent falls as a result, which of course can lead to serious injury. If a person who falls is living at home with an aged caregiver, it may not be possible for the caregiver to pick the person up, and 911 must be called. Again, this scenario frequently leads to placement in a long-term care facility—someone falls and is on the floor for a prolonged period of time (injured or not) while assistance is sought to help them get up. Falls occur, of course, in nursing homes as well, and can lead to serious injury; but at least there are staff present who can get someone off the floor.

B Is for Behavior

It is estimated that at least 90% of patients will have one or more significant mood or behavioral problems during the course of the illness. The most common behavioral symptoms in Alzheimer's disease are the following:

- Apathy
- Depression
- Anxiety
- Irritability
- Delusions
- Hallucinations
- Sleep disturbance
- Agitation
- Aggression
- Restlessness
- Anxiety
- Disinhibition

These are not separate psychiatric illnesses that happen to occur in persons with Alzheimer's but are a regular component of the disease itself. This is why it is useful to think of Alzheimer's as a neuropsychiatric illness, rather than simply a medical or neurologic condition.

Behavioral problems are understandably one of the most significant causes of stress for caregivers. Dealing with behavioral problems can wear out the sturdiest caregiver. Behavioral difficulties—particularly agitation in its various forms—along with bowel incontinence are the symptoms most likely to lead directly to nursing home placement. Because of their importance for the caregiver, mood and behavioral issues in Alzheimer's disease are discussed separately in Chapter 7.

C Is for Cognition

Cognitive symptoms are the hallmark of Alzheimer's disease. The cognitive domains that can be impaired are as follows:

1. Memory impairment (amnesia)
2. Language disturbance (aphasia)
3. Difficulty carrying out motor tasks despite intact motor abilities (apraxia)
4. The inability to recognize people or places that should be familiar (agnosia)
5. Difficulties with planning, initiating, or organizing, and problems in social judgment (executive dysfunction)

Amnesia

The memory impairment that is most characteristic of Alzheimer's disease (and most other dementias) affects recent memory. Individuals—at least until late in the disease—are able to register information, or immediately recall it. That is to say, a person with mild or moderate Alzheimer's disease can usually repeat a few words or a simple phrase immediately afterward. But these words become subject to what is referred to as rapid forgetting and after a few minutes' delay can no longer be recalled. This impairment in recent memory is often the first symptom noted by family members, and one of the most prominent early in the disease. It is the cause of the repetitive comments or questions that can be so stressful for caregivers. The person does not recall having previously made a particular comment or asking a question, or does not remember the answer. Repetitiveness appears to increase when the subject is one that causes anxiety. As the disease progresses, the period of time when general events can be recalled becomes progressively shorter. Curiously, events from long ago may be remembered until quite late in the disease, particularly if they are especially meaningful, such as one's wedding, graduation from college, and so forth. For some caregivers, the fact that memories from years ago are recalled while events of the last few minutes or hours are forgotten is seen as counterintuitive, and the caregiver may feel that the individual is simply not trying hard enough or is using selective memory—that is, choosing to remember certain things while forgetting the rest. Occasionally people with Alzheimer's who are defensive about memory impairments will say that they forget intentionally, remembering only the things they want or need to remember. This is a defensive comment, designed to help people feel more in control of this frightening process.

As the disease progresses, more and more aspects of the past are forgotten, to the point where a woman married for 50 years may forget her married name and only recall her maiden name; eventually that may be lost as well, along with many of the basic historical facts of her life that make her who she is. In this way, people with Alzheimer's disease gradually lose their sense of personal identity.

Aphasia

Aphasia in Alzheimer's disease refers not to the sudden loss of language abilities, which may happen after a stroke that affects the speech area, but to a more gradual decline of language abilities as the disease progresses. This may begin with occasional difficulty coming up with someone's name. In fact, this is a common symptom of aging in otherwise normal persons at midlife and beyond. In Alzheimer's, however, the loss of names becomes more and more pronunced, and other proper nouns begin to be lost as well. As this condition progresses, other common words are lost or are used incorrectly. The individual may refer to "that thing you sit on" instead of saying "chair" or will refer to wearing a "clock" or a "timer" rather than a wristwatch. At this stage, the language difficulties may be quite apparent, but generally the caregiver (assuming that is a family member or someone who knows the individual very well) is able to discern what the person is attempting to say, although others who are less familiar with the person may have more difficulty. After a period of time, language may become so disordered that it either conveys very little information ("empty speech") or makes little, if any, sense. This is a source of enormous frustration for both the person with Alzheimer's disease and the caregiver, although at times the person with the disease does not seem aware that he or she is not speaking coherently. Eventually, most people with Alzheimer's disease will end up with very little if any coherent speech, or speech may be limited to a few over-learned phrases (e.g., "I'm fine; how are you?") or to profanities. Of course, as in all aspects of this disease, there is significant variability from person to person. Some remain fairly verbal until quite late in the disease, but others lose speech as an early manifestation of the disease.

Curiously, persons who have learned English as a second language will often revert to their native tongue, either completely or intermingled with English, while their language abilities are deteriorating. This can be true if someone has spoken English exclusively for many decades. Once people with Alzheimer's revert completely to their native tongue, speakers of that language will often say that their communications in the native tongue are not terribly coherent either, so this clearly represents a breakdown of the process of language use rather than simply the loss of English words.

People generally maintain a greater ability to understand language than to produce it. Occasionally, people will talk in front of someone who has Alzheimer's disease as if the person is not present, particularly if she cannot speak very coherently. It is important to remember that the individual may understand much more than she appears to, and feelings can easily be hurt. On the other hand, it is also important to keep in mind that the individual who has difficulty speaking may also have difficulty understanding what is being said. Communication is discussed in detail in Chapter 5.

Apraxia

Apraxia involves the loss of the ability to perform a particular movement or series of movements, despite having the desire and the physical ability to do so. In simple terms, the brain has a problem telling the muscles how to carry out a certain action. Apraxia leads directly to impairments in ADLs and is a good example of how the various domains of impairment—A, B, and C—are so intertwined with each other. The desire and intent to carry out the activity remain, but the cognitive ability—not the motor ability—to do so is lacking. Apraxia may be involved in some failures of IADLs as well, such as not being able to place a letter or a check in an envelope, seal the envelope, and put a stamp on it. As apraxia worsens, much that has been taken for granted becomes lost, and the individual needs increasing amounts of support with simple tasks. Caregivers sometimes do not understand how this can be a function of dementia, particularly if, for example, yesterday or even earlier today the person could eat with his fork, but by dinnertime this skill seems to have been lost. As with so many of the impairments in Alzheimer's disease, there is great variability from person to person, from one day to the next, and from one time of day to another.

Agnosia

Agnosia causes the person with Alzheimer's disease to be unable to recognize people, places, or objects that should be familiar. This is not a visual problem per se; it has to do with recognition of what is clearly seen. This is different, of course, from seeing someone you know and not being able to think of her name. You may know lots of facts about this person but simply cannot retrieve the "label," either at all or at the moment it is called for. This is an anomia (a type of aphasia), not an agnosia. Gradually, agnosia worsens over time so that individuals who should be quite familiar to the person with Alzheimer's—neighbors, more distant relatives—are not recognized. Eventually, immediate family members are included—perhaps starting with children who live out of town and visit less frequently, but ultimately involving not recognizing the primary caregiver, even if it is the spouse of many decades. Understandably, this is most upsetting for the spouse, but it is also upsetting for the person with Alzheimer's, who may feel that there is a stranger in the house. As the process of agnosia is beginning, the individual with Alzheimer's may have some sense that someone is familiar but cannot be exactly identified. Or the nature of the relationship may become confused; a spouse is seen as a mother or father, an adult son as a brother.

Occasionally, the individual may be certain that his spouse, for example, is not around but has been replaced by someone who looks a little or a lot like her, who may even have the same name. This seems to represent an incomplete loss of recognition of the individual, but can be very confusing to all concerned. At times the person with Alzheimer's may feel that the person who lives with him is not his spouse (indeed, he may no longer recall that he was ever married) but will feel that this person is a very good friend.

As these agnosias are developing, they can be transient, so that someone may not recognize her spouse at one moment but a few minutes later will be able to identify him correctly. It may be possible for an unrecognized spouse to merely leave the room for a few moments and return, and then be recognized. At other times, an individual may not recognize his wife visually but, when she speaks, will be able to use the combination of auditory and visual stimuli to correctly identify her.

Occasionally, a person with dementia will be unable to recognize his own image in a mirror or a photograph. When this happens, he may believe that there is an intruder in his home. Eventually, all of the mirrors in the house may need to be removed or covered, and it may be important to ensure that the curtains are drawn before dark, so that the image reflected in the glass is not seen as someone prowling around outside the home.

Agnosia occurs not only in regard to people but for places as well. Someone with dementia may lose the ability to recognize her own house and insist on going home, which can lead to wandering, as she may go out the door and down the street, looking for home. At times, these persons seem to have in mind a home where they lived earlier in life, but that is not always the case. Occasionally, the individual will seem to partially recognize her home, feeling that this house looks very similar to her house but is different. Sometimes, persons with this sort of partial agnosia can be reoriented by gently pointing out that it is, indeed, their house, but perhaps it doesn't look quite the same "in this light" or something of the sort. Most of the time, however, people with these mistaken beliefs due to agnosias cannot be persuaded through the force of logic, and trying to do so will only upset them.

Disturbance of Executive Function

Executive function involves two broad areas of concern. One has to do with the ability to initiate behaviors, to maintain them, and to terminate them when appropriate. This includes the ability to know how to sequence steps to accomplish a task. The other area of concern has to do with judgment: that is, knowing—and caring—what is appropriate behavior in a given social or interpersonal context. It also involves being able to make accurate judgments of people and situations to protect one's own interests.

Initiation

Individuals with deficits in executive function often have difficulty initiating behavior. This is directly related to apathy, a prominent feature of Alzheimer's disease and other dementias, which is discussed in more detail in Chapter 7.

Many people who are able, perhaps with help, to initiate an activity are unable to follow the necessary steps to its conclusion. This leads directly to impairments in functioning. Being able to follow the correct sequence of steps to review a bill, write out a check properly, enter the check stub information correctly, address the envelope, put a stamp on it, and mail it is an example of a complex sequence of behaviors that requires executive ability, and one that is frequently impaired even in early Alzheimer's disease. Another breakdown of proper sequencing coming somewhat later in the disease would involve being unable to follow the correct steps to get dressed in the morning, even with all of the clothes laid out on the bed. This can lead to significant frustration on the part of the individual who is trying to get dressed and can also be quite stressful for the caregiver when it becomes necessary to dress the person entirely. This is a good example of how the various domains of impairment interact inseparably—cognitive impairments lead directly to difficulties in functioning, which cause frustration and possibly more overt expressions of anger or aggressiveness, which in turn lead to greater stress and burden for the caregiver. It is really only possible to separate A, B, C, and D artificially, for the sake of discussion, since they are so intertwined in reality.

Judgment

The other critical area of executive functioning involves judgment, which requires a number of high-level cognitive tasks and thus is often impaired in subtle or not-so-subtle ways early in the course of disease. Impairments in social and interpersonal judgment lead directly to a wide range of behavioral problems and conflicts with others, while impairments in the ability to correctly judge other people and situations can make someone vulnerable to exploitation. Again, these are somewhat artificial distinctions for the sake of discussion, but they are certainly interrelated areas of concern, perhaps two sides of the same coin.

A number of the behavioral problems discussed in Chapter 7 may occur because of lack of social appropriateness. Thus, someone who is unable to perform a given task might not simply feel some sense of frustration internally, but might become quite angry, possibly verbally abusive, in response. This type of overreaction has been referred to as the "catastrophic reaction" by Mace and Rabins (1999) in *The 36-Hour Day*. It is a very useful way of understanding some of the emotional storms that seemingly come from nowhere, or in response to minor stressors. Individuals who react this way are unable to recognize and carry out the socially appropriate response to a given situation; and they may also be unable to stop the reaction due to their executive dysfunction.

Other examples of impaired social judgment include patients who curse in settings where they might never have done that before, or make off-color or bigoted remarks in the presence of those who would be offended. Persons with more advanced disease in nursing homes may walk in the halls undressed, masturbate publicly, make sexually inappropriate comments to staff, or make unwanted sexual advances to staff or other residents.

It is sometimes impossible to tell if the individual does not recognize that a given behavior is offensive to others, or if she knows that others are offended but does not feel any concern about that. This lack of awareness or concern for the feelings of others leads some to view the person with Alzheimer's as self-centered, unkind, or even somewhat sociopathic. These labels certainly lead to a great deal of negative feelings toward the individual and do not help with managing the situation. It is important for the clinician to help family members see that these behaviors, as distasteful as they may be, are symptoms of the illness rather than willful or morally corrupt behaviors. This awareness may help control the caregiver's anger and lead to more appropriate ways of dealing with the situation.

Vulnerability to Exploitation

Occasionally, a person first comes to the attention of family or professionals because he or she has been the victim of exploitation. Usually, this is financial, but it can occur in other domains as well. Other common exploitations involve hired caregiving help who ask to "borrow" money or say they need $100 to buy some items for the person at the grocery store, when all they are getting is a few staples. Other individuals find themselves giving money to every charity that sends them junk mail, some of which are certainly legitimate while others are not; or entering sweepstakes that promise huge prizes if only the person will buy certain magazine subscriptions. Unfortunately, signing up for one uncertain scheme or one dubious charity only ensures that much more junk mail will be coming soon. Persons who would have thrown away junk mail without thinking about it in the past may now spend much of the day going through it all and responding to it because of the clever but nefarious sales techniques of the senders. Many families find they simply need to make sure they get to the mail-box before the person with dementia, tossing out much of what arrives.

Now that increasing numbers of older individuals are computer literate (although it usually diminishes with increasing dementia), there is a parallel concern about junk e-mails and the many scams that daily arrive in one's e-mail inbox. Persons with mild Alz-heimer's disease can spend tens of thousands of dollars in these pursuits. Some of this has to do with not remembering or keeping good track of what was previously purchased; and much of it has to do with not being able to exercise good judgment in the face of sales pressures. Unfortunately, there is no shortage of unscrupu-lous individuals who are aware of the judgment difficulties of many older individuals and stand ready to prey on them merci-lessly. One of the most important tasks of caregivers of persons with even very early Alzheimer's disease is to set up safeguards to protect the person with diminished judgment from being ex-ploited. It is important for the clinician to warn family members that, even though the person with dementia had previously exer-cised excellent judgment, that ability can become significantly im-paired even in the early stages of the illness.

STAGES OF THE ILLNESS

Alzheimer's disease is a progressive illness. From diagnosis (often several years after symptoms have begun) until death, any-where from 2 to 20 years can elapse. The typical person with Alzheimer's has symptoms for about 10 years from diagnosis to death, although that depends on numerous factors such as the per-son's age at the time of onset, general health, the quality and in-tensity of medical care throughout the disease, and so forth.

With or without treatment the disease progresses relentlessly from onset until the time of death. It is therefore useful to talk about stages of illness, just as cancer, heart disease, and other long-term illnesses are often staged. It is important to remember, however, that there is great variability from one individual to the next in Alzheimer's, and while certain characteristics may be typical of a person at, say, the moderate stage of the disease, features of more advanced illness as well as more mild symptoms may be present. Staging is useful for clinicians and others, as a shorthand, to communicate some information about a given person without having to describe all of the things that they can still do or no longer do. But staging is only a rough approximation.

The most common staging system is the simple three-stage system. People with Alzheimer's are classified as having either mild, moderate, or severe disease. In practice, specialists also speak frequently of persons with mild-to-moderate or moderate-to-severe disease, when features of both stages are present; the term end-stage disease refers to the final substage of severe dementia.

Mild Stage

Typical features of mild or early-stage Alzheimer's disease include the following:

- Impairment of recent memory begins to impact day-to-day life.
- Disorientation to time, place common.
- Loss of initiative (apathy).
- Mood and personality changes may occur.
- Impairment of judgment in decision making.
- Difficulty managing money, paying bills, and so on (IADLs).

To qualify for a diagnosis of Alzheimer's disease (or other dementia) as opposed to MCI, there needs to be evidence that the impairments have an impact on daily life. This is a gray area that can be difficult to determine. For example, just how much difficulty remembering names is beyond the boundaries of MCI and qualifies instead for a diagnosis of Alzheimer's? While one never makes the diagnosis purely on the basis of one symptom category, impairment in daily functioning is present if someone refuses to go to social events or to lunches at the senior center because they can no longer reliably remember anyone's name there. Another example of memory impairment beginning to affect daily life might be someone who becomes toxic from taking his daily medications twice, or not at all for several days in a row, or makes other significant medication errors.

Because of these difficulties, persons with mild Alzheimer's disease generally need some supervision or assistance from others on a daily basis. Usually, however, they are able to live in the community with family, or even alone with sufficient, regular caregiver support and assistance.

Moderate Stage

Persons with moderate-stage disease typically display the following characteristics:

- Increasing memory loss and confusion
- Difficulty recognizing friends and family (usually not spouse or primary caregiver, although this varies)
- Significant difficulty with reading, writing, and finding words
- Loss of impulse control
- Reluctance or refusal to bathe
- Difficulty with dressing and other ADLs, without need of total assistance with these
- Significant mood or behavioral problems

Moderate-stage Alzheimer's covers a wide range of functions and impairments. Someone in the early-moderate stages of disease may need some help with cueing to get dressed, whereas someone in the late-moderate stages may need near total assistance with ADLs. Similarly, speech may be only mildly disturbed, or it may be almost completely incoherent. Because of the wide range of impairments, people with moderate disease may live at home, with considerable help from caregivers. Usually, they do not live alone unless someone is assisting them for at least some period of time every day, and that is not an ideal situation in most cases. Other individuals with moderate dementia may reside in a memory care unit of an assisted living facility, or possibly even a nursing home, depending on their degree of dependency or concurrent medical problems.

Severe Stage

By the time individuals reach the severe stages of Alzheimer's, they usually have been ill for many years. Typical symptoms at this stage include:

- Little or no short-term memory.
- Complete assistance with all basic ADLs is needed.
- Language is extremely impaired, if still present; it is difficult or impossible to understand communications in either direction (i.e., expressive and receptive).
- Usually incontinent of both urine and bowel.

Individuals in the severe stage of dementia are frequently in a nursing home, due to their impairment in all ADLs and incontinence. If they are still living at home, they need continuous care for survival as they are literally unable to do anything for themselves.

End Stage

The final phase of severe dementia is referred to as the end stage. Persons in end-stage dementia often show the following characteristics:

- Weight loss; increasing difficulty with eating or reluctance to eat
- Inability to recognize even close family members
- Minimal or no language
- Minimal to no interaction with the environment; automatic reactions only to being stimulated

End-stage dementia is discussed in greater detail in Chapter 10.

CHAPTER 3

Facing the Problem

As noted earlier, people frequently suffer for several years with symptoms of Alzheimer's disease before a diagnosis is finally made and treatment is begun, for a number of reasons: the gradual onset of the disease, the subtlety of early symptoms, and the time and expertise needed for a busy physician to take the necessary history and perform office tests. However, two other issues play a very important role in contributing to this delay: the stigma associated with Alzheimer's disease and other memory disorders, and denial in the person with Alzheimer's disease, as well as the Alzheimer's family.

THE STIGMA OF ALZHEIMER'S DISEASE

One of the great burdens of Alzheimer's disease is the stigma that families and society as a whole feel about it. Fortunately, the disease has gradually become more public, beginning perhaps with Ronald Reagan's admission that he was suffering from the disease shortly after completing his presidency, and thanks to his and his family's regular public statements about his status throughout his illness. Nevertheless, many are quite uncomfortable—or worse, ashamed—to talk about having the condition themselves or having a loved one with it. Some view it as "moral weakness," just as some view mental illness this way. If only the person "tried harder," he would remember better.

From the earliest years in school, students are taught that to remember more is better and will earn them better grades. While most educators would say that learning should be more than just rote memorization, nevertheless much of educational structure and rewards are based on how well one can recall what has been taught. From the earliest years through college and graduate school, students are rewarded with good grades for remembering facts well. Conversely, getting poor grades on a test that involves memorization means the individual did not study enough or may not be very bright. Poor memory therefore is associated with being lazy or unintelligent or both. This is certainly one contributor to the negative connotations associated with the impaired remembering of Alzheimer's disease. Many of my patients talk about "failing" memory tests given by Alzheimer's specialists, and some will even "cram" before an appointment, wanting to do well, as if the cognitive examination were a quiz in high school physics or history. Occasionally, a family member or the person suffering with Alzheimer's will try to excuse errors with comments such as, "He doesn't know what day it is because we didn't get a chance to look at the paper today before coming here" or something similar.

It would appear that people (members of the general public, but also some health care providers, and sometimes even members of the Alzheimer's family) have a different view of illnesses that involve frailties of the body compared to those which involve frailties of the mind. Even though it could be argued that the mind is nothing more than the conscious manifestation of processes occurring in the brain, special significance is attached to disorders of the mind. A broken leg is fundamentally different in the thinking of most people than a broken mind. As noted above, there appears to be a feeling—even among those who should know better—that a person with a broken leg cannot help it, but someone with Alzheimer's disease is somehow at least partially responsible for the problem. The same stigma applies as well to certain mental illnesses such as depression, schizophrenia, and the like. While these stigmas have lessened somewhat in recent years, they are still very much present. Stigma, after all, is a way of labeling people and having a set of preconceived feelings about them that are not based on direct knowledge of the person involved. In that sense, it is a form of prejudice or bias.

People with Alzheimer's are victimized by this prejudice in a great many ways. They are seen as different; deficient somehow and frightening at times. They are "them" while the people who do not have Alzheimer's disease are "us." These prejudices exist in senior communities where those with Alzheimer's disease or other dementias live among those who do not. Those with Alzheimer's—and often their spouses—may not be invited to community activities. In communal dining settings, people tend to avoid sitting with those who have the disease. As a result, the individual and the spouse often dine alone together in a dining room full of people enjoying each other's company. When people approach a couple, one of whom has the disease, they will often speak to the nonafflicted individual, ignoring the person with the disease as if he or she is not present or is completely incapable of understanding what is being said or responding appropriately. At other times, people will speak to the individual with the disease in a demeaning, overly simplified way, with vocal inflections and patterns similar to the way people speak to children.

Behind these behavioral slights and insults is ignorance, certainly, and perhaps an innocent concern about not saying or doing something that might upset the individual with the disease. These behaviors—particularly avoidance of the person with Alzheimer's disease—may also represent fear on the part of nonafflicted elders who have great apprehension about developing dementia themselves. Dealing with a strong fear by simply avoiding the source is a common defense mechanism.

People with Alzheimer's disease remain quite attuned to the nonverbal messages given by others—perhaps they are even more attuned to nonverbal cues than before, since they can no longer rely on verbal memory and other aspects of cognition to help understand their relationship with other people. The awareness, on some level, of being different than others further worsens the already low self-esteem that is common among those with Alzheimer's, particularly early in the process. And it contributes to the loss of the sense of self of the person afflicted.

In a similar way, those who associate with the stigmatized person—the Alzheimer's family, primarily—become stigmatized themselves. They become identified by their relationship with the afflicted person and less as individuals in their own right. This is, of course, most true for the primary caregiver, and less so for other members of the Alzheimer's family.

DENIAL

Denial is a multifaceted concept. The stigma of the disease certainly contributes to denial in Alzheimer's, but there is much more involved.

Denial is an unconscious thought process in which one lessens anxiety by refusing to acknowledge the existence of specific unpleasant aspects of external reality or of one's own thoughts or feelings. In common usage, denial often refers to the activity of someone who is not acknowledging the existence of something that is plainly obvious to others. Often there is the implication that this is intentional, akin to concealment, covering up, or even lying. Thus it often has a pejorative or negative connotation and is seen as willful rather than as an unconscious defense mechanism employed by everyone to a greater or lesser degree. In fact, denial can be very helpful in maintaining mental and emotional equanimity; it can help preserve self-esteem, decrease anxiety, and avoid a sense of hopelessness and despair. Denial is a vital defense mechanism that allows us to (unconsciously) control how much bad news we must face and when. For example, the person who is diagnosised with an advanced cancer that is often fatal in a short period of time may hold onto the notion that he or she will be able to beat the odds, respond to chemotherapy, and go into indefinite remission. Gradually, as reality sets in, the person may realize that is unlikely and, as symptoms increase, eventually face the reality that the disease is going to be fatal. Facing all of this at once would be overwhelming, and it is very understandable that someone would unconsciously incorporate this terrible news only gradually.

On the other hand, excessive denial can become destructive or even fatal. For example, a woman who for many months ignores a lump in her breast, telling herself it is probably nothing, until the lesion grows through the skin and serious systemic symptoms develop, may have permitted the cancer to spread and become incurable because of the delay in seeking medical attention, due to her denial. All doctors know how common this scenario is. Thus, there is healthy denial and pathological denial. Individuals—and families—who ignore the signs of memory impairment for months, rationalizing that they are due to aging, fatigue, poor hearing, or laziness, so that an evaluation and diagnosis are delayed by many months, or longer, may be allowing the disease to progress significantly before treatment is instituted. This may not have the same fatal consequences as ignoring a serious breast lump, but many adverse events can occur that might be avoided if the disease is recognized, diagnosed, and treated as soon as symptoms appear.

In most cases, the denial of the individual with cognitive impairment is much greater than that of the family, but it is important to realize that the family's denial is a critical factor that determines when the afflicted person gets evaluated, and how openly he or she accepts the diagnosis and treatment offered. Whenever a family has significant denial, it can be almost impossible to persuade the person with Alzheimer's to accept the need for treatment, safety measures, and the like. Thus, the family's denial must be addressed first, often before it is possible to evaluate and treat the person with memory loss.

In addressing denial in the family, just as in the individual, it is important for the clinician to determine what unpleasant or frightening awareness is being avoided. How exactly does the possibility of Alzheimer's disease most upset the family equilibrium? Of course, it upsets it in every possible way; but what are the most concerning issues for the family? It usually is important to explore these issues with the family, usually without the afflicted person present, as it is quite unlikely that family members will express their fears in front of the person with Alzheimer's. Discussing specific areas of concern in detail, rather than simply saying that the whole situation is terrible, is helpful for the family to face their specific fears about the disease. Facing it and talking about it in this way can lessen family denial. Of course it does not help to say, "It's not that bad"—it *is* "that bad," and worse. For example, if the afflicted individual will not be able to drive, and no one else at home drives, that reality must be acknowledged, but then time needs to be spent in trying to solve this new problem: who can help with driving; how errands can be accomplished; what public transportation exists; and what to do with the car, for example. This is not done to diminish the severity of this new reality; it is merely to explore methods to begin to cope with it.

Of course, the greatest reason for denial in a family member, particularly a spouse or adult child, is to avoid or diminish the realization that a diagnosis marks the beginning of the loss of the person with Alzheimer's disease. The afflicted person is no longer who he or she used to be, and rather than being a temporary aberration, the situation will get inexorably worse. Along with giving up significant elements of their denial comes an acknowledgment of the family's need to begin to relinquish—to say goodbye—to the person with the disease. Helping the family face their grief and work through the accompanying emotions of sadness, anxiety, anger, guilt, and—finally—acceptance may be the most important single task of the clinician working with a member of the Alzheimer's family.

The process of working through denial is gradual. It is never the case that denial is present today, worked through, and gone tomorrow, either for the family or the individual with the disease. There may be denial about each aspect of loss, each new area of impairment, each new stage of disease. Denial can lessen and then grow strong again in the face of new anxieties. Dealing with denial should be viewed as an ongoing process, not as a single obstacle that has to be addressed, removed, and forgotten. It is most helpful, in this process, for the clinician to assist the family to reach a considerable degree of awareness of the nature of the disease, along with a genuine acceptance that it is better for them, and for the person with Alzheimer's, to face the situation realistically than to try to continue to deny or avoid it.

In most cases, the family will be the chief agent of change for the afflicted person's denial—more so, generally, than the physician. While the physician may be the expert and the figure of authority, he or she is seen only intermittently by the person with the disease, and communications from the physician are often forgotten between visits. It is the family's constant (or very frequent) presence that helps lessen denial and increase acceptance of the disease by the afflicted person. This is certainly not accomplished by insisting that the individual "admit" he or she has Alzheimer's disease, but by adopting the attitude described above—that facing the situation realistically, as painful as it may be, is better for everyone than continuing to deny, avoid, or minimize it. Some persons who suffer from the disease are reasonably able to accept this, once the family has reached this point. Other individuals need to maintain a significant degree of denial throughout the illness. While this certainly makes it more difficult for the family to care for the person, it may be difficult or impossible to significantly lessen that denial until the individual is somehow ready to do so.

It is also important to keep in mind the difference between denial in words and denial in behavior. For example, it is often critical that the person with Alzheimer's agree not to drive. The individual may not acknowledge that his or her driving is dangerous because of cognitive difficulties. It may be much easier to say that driving is becoming dangerous because of poor vision or some other physical ailment. What is important is to end the driving, not to insist that the person acknowledge that this has to do with Alzheimer's. That awareness may simply not exist, or the individual may feel too great a sense of shame (due to stigma) over the loss of cognitive abilities. In other words, what is critical is what the individual does, not what he or she says. As long as certain basic steps are taken to provide for safety and appropriate treatment, the reasons the person gives for his or her behavior are less critical. That is not because the family should be indifferent to this, but because they respect the individual enough to permit him or her to maintain a degree of denial, in order to maintain self-esteem, as long as the right things are done.

THE FAMILY INTERVENTION FOR SEVERE DENIAL

The intensity of denial in a person with Alzheimer's may be so great and so persistent, over time, that the situation becomes worrisome, or even dangerous. The individual may adamantly refuse to have an evaluation despite significant impairments in cognition, which are worsening steadily. Or it may be that an individual who is no longer driving safely refuses to consider limiting or giving up driving. Difficult behavioral issues may develop such as paranoia, irritability, or agitation.

The person with Alzheimer's disease who is so firmly in denial may be someone who has always needed to be in control—a so-called Type A personality. These individuals are found in every walk of life, but are common among executives, physicians, attorneys, and other careers where being in charge is part of one's identity. Type As are frequently, but not exclusively, male. This intense denial also occurs in persons who have been widowed or divorced relatively early in life, and have been on their own—and often fiercely independent—for decades.

People who have extreme difficulty accepting that something is wrong cognitively are not just control freaks who enjoy being difficult but are generally people whose self-esteem is extremely dependent on being in full control of themselves at all times. It therefore takes a great deal of sensitivity to confront denial in this sort of person, and it is important to recognize that they are quite vulnerable to becoming depressed (which they may also deny, intensely) once there is some breakdown in their denial about their cognitive difficulties.

When individual family efforts to get the person to accept the need for care or supervision fail, it may be necessary to plan an intervention. An intervention to address cognitive issues is similar to that which is sometimes necessary with a person who is alcoholic but refuses to accept any assistance or to consider stopping drinking. In both cases, strong denial is at work, but perhaps for different reasons.

The intervention to address denial should occur when family members have come to feel that the situation is becoming untenable and dangerous. Interventions can be difficult, emotionally, for all concerned, and can backfire if feelings get out of control. It may be advisable for the clinician to meet with members of the family (without the person with cognitive difficulties) to discuss the specifics of the situation and to offer advice on how to conduct this delicate operation. It may be that the clinician will recommend that the intervention take place after working with a member of the Alzheimer's family and hearing about how difficult the situation is becoming.

Family members often feel that they have no right to talk about a member of the family behind his back; or that they are being disloyal to the person with cognitive problems if they talk to others and do not include the afflicted individual. While these sentiments are understandable, it may be helpful for the clinician to point out that there is nothing loyal in allowing someone's illness to go unchecked, worsening over time. In fact it is a most loyal act to get a loved one the help he or she needs, even if the very illness from which the individual suffers interferes with the recognition of that need. Talking to a clinician about the problem, without the person present (because it might well be impossible to discuss it openly otherwise) should therefore be viewed as an act of love, not disloyalty. The clinician will have to assist the family with this cognitive reframing, as it seems to go against long-held values.

The clinician may need to help the family members examine and adjust their view of their relationship to the person with cognitive difficulties in other ways, as well. They may believe that the afflicted person is too powerful to confront or, alternatively, too fragile. Neither is likely to be true. They may feel intimidated by the anger that may well result from the intervention. It may be important for the clinician to assess the likelihood of physical aggressiveness. If that appears to be a serious risk, then no intervention should occur without appropriate measures to ensure the safety of all concerned.

Perhaps the most important reason for hesitation on the family's part is their uncertainty about how to express their concerns to the afflicted individual without insulting him or causing needless hurt and distress. This is, indeed, the essence of the matter, the main reason that interventions can be so difficult. In general, it is best for family members to focus on concrete examples of the individual's behavior (e.g., pointing out that he has not taken necessary heart medications on more days than not this past month or has put four new scrapes in the car in the last few months) rather than making general statements that can be seen as judgmental (e.g., "You are becoming very forgetful" or "You have become a dangerous driver"). The concerns should be presented in a matter-of-fact and not guilt-provoking manner. And for every comment that could be seen as a criticism, there needs to be emphasis on the individual's preserved abilities and the family's affection and respect for the person in spite of whatever difficulties are present. For example, it may be helpful to say, "But we really love how you have such a wonderful ability to recall the old days. We'd really like to record some of your great stories from when you were young."

While the clinician can be very helpful to the family in preparing for the intervention, confronting the afflicted person is a job for those who know him best. Generally, the spouse (if there is a living spouse) and adult children should be present for the intervention. If there are no children, or none nearby, the situation is obviously more difficult. This is not something that can successfully be done over the telephone—it must occur in person. When no children are available, other relatives who have a close relationship with the individual, such as a sibling, might then participate. It may also include a close personal friend or a priest or minister.

The intervention should be scheduled at a time of day when the individual generally is at his best, cognitively, which often means in the morning. Those present should be available for at least a couple of hours; it is important that those present stay and participate for the entire intervention. And most critically, all present should be on the same page in regard to the seriousness of the problem and the need to do something about it. No matter how many people are present, if there is just one family member or friend who sides with the afflicted person in feeling that too much is being made of the problem, or that it is really not as bad as everyone else believes, the person with Alzheimer's will somehow only hear that person's point of view (even if he is mostly quiet during the intervention) and the process will have been traumatic but not successful.

Generally no more than four or five family members or friends should be present for the intervention; anything more than that will be too confusing and will increase the discomfort of the afflicted person. It should generally occur in the afflicted person's own home, and never in a public setting.

The spouse or other close relative is generally the one who should take the lead unless that individual is too fearful of the process and the potential reaction. In that case, it should be someone who can firmly inform the afflicted person what the concerns are, without anger but also without backing down when the inevitable denial and anger start to be expressed by the person with Alzheimer's. As noted above, it can be a delicate matter to make the intervention forceful without the afflicted person feeling that his loved ones are ganging up on him. In fact, they are ganging up, but it must be repeated, over and over, that it is being done out of love, and out of concern, and out of the strong feeling that something needs to be done. It will be important—but difficult—not to argue with the confronted person, because that individual will likely find factual errors or alternate explanations for some if not all of the incidents being described. Even if the family is convinced of the accuracy of their version of every incident described, the point should be made that it is the sum of all of these events, and others, that leads to the concerns, and not any single event.

The goal of the confrontation, as with denial in general, is not to force the individual to admit to having cognitive problems, but to agree to take certain actions, whether or not he agrees they are necessary. So it is critical to determine, before beginning the intervention, what concrete actions will be asked of the person. Perhaps it is to give up driving, one of the more difficult sacrifices a person can be asked to make (see Chapter 6). Perhaps it is to accept having a paid caregiver come to the house when other family members are not available. Perhaps it is merely to go for an evaluation or take antidementia medication that has already been prescribed but refused. It may be necessary to emphasize that the individual is being asked to do this for the family, because it will make the spouse or the family as a whole more comfortable, even if the afflicted individual does not personally feel the action is really necessary. Again, the goal is to change behavior, not to extract a confession about having Alzheimer's disease. That would be helpful, if it occurs as an insight that has happened as a result of the confrontation, but it is rare, unfortunately, at least at this point.

It is important to stress throughout that the intervention is being done because of the love and high esteem in which the person is held; it is not for punitive reasons, as it is often experienced. It is also helpful to point out that the goal of getting into some treatment (if that is the goal) is not because the person is deficient and needs to be "fixed" but, instead, to help the person maintain all of the abilities he now has for as long as possible. Sometimes a statement to the effect, "You are doing well and we just want to do all we can to keep it that way" can be useful, because it focuses on the abilities and strengths of the person, rather than the deficiencies. This might be a time when a "fiblet" (see Chapter 5) or a minor white lie is felt to be appropriate, because it is genuinely for the good of the afflicted individual. In reality, he may not be doing well at all, but the overall message is more likely to be accepted when these positive statements are included; and it is certainly true that the individual is doing better now than he will be in the future, particularly if no treatment is started.

Before the intervention concludes, it is very important that there be at least one point upon which everyone can agree. Even at the worst, if the afflicted individual will not agree to any change in his behavior, an attempt should be made to at least make an agreement that the entire issue will be revisited again, with another meeting, in a relatively short time.

It can be very helpful for someone present at the intervention to

write a brief summary of what has been discussed and (importantly) to what the afflicted person has agreed, whether or not he
is still able to comprehend and appreciate the written word. It
should include the current date and a specific date in the near future when the situation will be reviewed to ensure that the agreement has been carried out. This date and other minor details can
serve as a point of negotiation with the afflicted person; he may
want to delay whatever has been agreed upon and, if appropriate,
this should be accepted so that the person with Alzheimer's can
genuinely feel that he has had some say in the final agreement.
For example, the family may wish to insist that driving be stopped
immediately but may be willing to compromise such that driving
to the post office and back, only, can continue so long as it is not
raining or snowing, until the situation is reviewed again in a
month's time. This should be written up in 150 words or less and
signed by the person with Alzheimer's. Signed copies should be
made for everyone present, including two copies, at least, for the
person with Alzheimer's, with one posted in a prominent place,
such as the refrigerator. It is likely that the document will need to
be reviewed in the future. It is also possible that this type of intervention will need to occur more than once. A second (or third) intervention may be necessary if, in spite of the agreements reached
previously, no change has occurred. And if no progress has been
made, it would be valuable for the family to meet with the clinician to discuss how to proceed.

GETTING A DIAGNOSIS

While it is never good news to get a diagnosis of Alzheimer's
disease or other serious cognitive disorder, it is often a relief to individuals and families who have long suspected that something
was wrong but could not identify exactly what the problem was.

Getting a diagnosis also allows persons who are afflicted, and
their families, to begin to plan for the future, and for the person
with Alzheimer's disease (before cognition becomes too impaired)
to play an active role in that planning. It also allows steps to be
taken to ensure safety and to lessen the chance for exploitation of

the cognitively impaired individual. Getting a diagnosis of Alzheimer's disease should also encourage individuals to begin the process of completing advance directives as soon as possible, if it has not already been done. Waiting will risk that the person with Alzheimer's will progress to the point where he is no longer able to complete these documents legally.

Getting a diagnosis of Alzheimer's disease also gives the patient and family an opportunity to learn all they can about the disease, to better deal with it. Finally, getting a diagnosis can lead to the initiation of medication treatment, which may slow the rate of disease progression (see appendix).

As noted, the diagnostic process must begin with sufficient lessening of denial on the part of the individual and the family to recognize that something is wrong that needs to be investigated. The notion that becoming forgetful is an inevitable part of the aging process needs to be rejected. Individuals and families should not be led into thinking that it will get better with time; with time and without treatment memory disorders almost always get worse.

Getting a diagnosis should usually begin with an evaluation by the primary physician. It is essential that a member of the family or other care partner be part of that evaluation, as it is unlikely that a person with a memory disorder will be able to tell the physician everything needed to make a diagnosis. It is also unlikely that the person with a memory disorder will be able to remember enough of what went on in the visit with the doctor to be informative to the care partner. A physician who does not permit a care partner to be part of the diagnostic visit or who dismisses the concerns of the individual, stating, "It's normal to be forgetful when you get older" may be the wrong physician for the person with memory concerns, and another medical opinion should be sought. Fortunately, those attitudes are increasingly uncommon (but not unheard of) these days.

The evaluation by the primary physician may be limited or extensive, depending on the usual practice of that physician. Some primary care physicians are very skilled at diagnosing and treating persons with Alzheimer's disease or other memory disorders, while others prefer to refer all persons with these concerns to a specialist. When symptoms are atypical, rapidly progressive, not responding to appropriate treatment, or causing a great deal of distress, a specialist should definitely be consulted. That specialist might be a geriatrician, a neurologist, or a geriatric psychiatrist. The nature of the individual's symptoms may determine which specialist is needed. For example, if there are neurologic symptoms or the presentation has atypical features, a neurologist might be the appropriate specialist. If mood or behavioral difficulties are a particular concern, then a geriatric psychiatrist would be appropriate. In cases of significant medical comorbidity that may be contributing to the picture, such as diabetes, a geriatric internist would be the best option.

THE DIAGNOSTIC EVALUATION

The initial evaluation for Alzheimer's disease, particularly when performed in a specialty clinic or office, is an important opportunity for the person who is afflicted and for the family. The person with cognitive problems should simply be himself at the evaluation, but the family should actively prepare for the meeting, to get the most out of the visit.

Generally, it is a good idea for the primary caregiver and at most one other family member to be present during the evaluation interview of the afflicted person. It is not helpful to have a large number of family members present, which can be distracting to the person being evaluated and to the evaluator. Families should decide ahead of time who will be the family spokesperson or persons, and every family member's information about the afflicted individual should be funneled through the spokesperson.

In some memory clinics, the person with cognitive issues is interviewed alone, while another clinician, often a social worker, sees the family separately. However, people with cognitive disorders are generally more comfortable having their primary caregiver in the room when they are being interviewed. Others prefer to be seen alone, and if some degree of tension is noted, it may be appropriate for the family members to wait in the waiting room. This may be especially true when the cognitive examination is performed. However, it may be useful for the family to witness the individual's performance on the cognitive test. Whether or not the primary caregiver is present for some of or the entire initial interview, the evaluating physician will usually see the afflicted person alone for part of the interview. Generally it can make it difficult for the person with cognitive problems to feel comfortable with the physician if the physician also spends time with the family alone; this is why it is so valuable for the primary caregiver or other members of the family to establish a relationship with a clinician with whom they can work throughout the course of illness. Permission should be established from the beginning for the clinician and the physician to speak with each other. This does not eliminate the need for the primary caregiver to attend follow-up appointments with the physician; even if the physician sees the person with Alzheimer's alone initially, there should be time at the end of the visit for the physician to discuss his or her impressions and recommendations for ongoing care, and to answer any questions that the primary caregiver may have. Typical questions involve the projected course of the illness; what to tell other family and friends; how much, if any, outside assistance is needed at this point; whether or not to correct cognitive errors which occur; and the like.

The initial evaluation can be a lengthy process, and may not be completed in the limited time the typical physician allots for each patient visit. It may therefore be necessary for the initial evaluation to take place over a number of different visits. This may be preferable, in fact, to lessen the chance that the person being evaluated will become excessively tired or irritated by the process. When that happens, the quality and reliability of the information gathered diminishes significantly. It is also important to avoid creating an unpleasant situation for the person being evaluated, either by an excessively long assessment or an attitude that focuses on the individual's shortcomings.

What Information Is Useful for the Evaluation Process

Information presented by the family is absolutely essential in the evaluation of someone suspected of having Alzheimer's disease. The nature of the condition is such that, by definition, the person being evaluated is not able to be a fully reliable historian. Both denial and simple forgetfulness play a role in this, along with other factors. Individuals who go for an initial evaluation of memory problems without a family member are not likely to have a very useful experience at the physician's office. Prior to the evaluation, it is most helpful if the family members make notes about their concerns. It is most helpful to the evaluating physician if the particular concerning behaviors are described, rather than simply indicating that the person has "forgetfulness" or "inappropriateness" or the like. It is important, as well, to know when these concerning behaviors began, even though in the typical case of Alzheimer's, the symptoms begin so gradually that it is often quite difficult to indicate the onset. In retrospect, families often realize that symptoms had been going on for some time. Some memory clinics may ask the family to complete a rather detailed questionnaire about the individual. The clinician working with the family can be particularly helpful by assisting with this. Whether or not there is a formal questionnaire, the information presented by the family should ideally be reviewed by the clinician to ensure that critical concerns are communicated to the memory clinic specialist. It is important for families to gather records of any previous cognitive evaluations, including brief memory tests or full neuropsychological test batteries. If neuroimaging scans of the brain have been performed (CT, MRI, or PET scan), the results of these tests, if not copies of the studies themselves, should certainly be forwarded to the clinic or brought in at the time of the evaluation. In the case of medications to help with memory or behavioral symptoms, the exact names and doses of the medications used, the duration of use of the medication, and any effects noted should be carefully compiled for the evaluating physician. Of course, current medications and doses should be clearly listed. What is actually being taken may be different from what the hospital or clinic record shows. Also, it is no longer helpful to the clinician to learn that someone takes a "small orange pill," because the common use of generics makes identifying medications by their shape and size almost impossible now.

The Chief Complaint

Most medical evaluations begin with a statement of the "chief complaint"—that is, what it is that brings the person to the memory specialist at this time. In the case of Alzheimer's disease, the individual may be at the evaluation only because he or she has acquiesced to the family's strong request for the evaluation. It is not uncommon to get as an answer to the question "What brings you here?" a mildly annoyed pointing of the finger at the family members present, and the answer, "*They* did." In such situations, the memory specialist will indicate that the person being evaluated has no particular complaints (if that continues to be the case) but that family members were concerned about forgetfulness, or getting lost, a personality change, hallucinations, or some other symptom or symptoms.

The History of the Present Illness

The detailed evaluation of someone with memory complaints involves taking a thorough history of the symptoms from both the patient and caregiver. It is important for the memory specialist to determine if the symptoms began gradually or suddenly. As noted earlier, in the case of the typical person with Alzheimer's disease, symptoms begin extremely gradually. Individuals and family members alike will often point to a particular event as the marker for the sudden beginning of the illness. The event may be an illness, a medical procedure, an accident, or some other stressor. While it may well be that symptoms worsened at the time of this stress, careful history will often reveal that symptoms were present for some time before the event, but perhaps had not reached a level of severity that could break through the denial, of all involved, and become noticeable.

It is natural for people to associate the onset of symptoms of an insidious illness like Alzheimer's with some external event, although that is usually not the case. However, symptoms do reach a tipping point, when a slight increase in symptom severity suddenly seems to change the individual from a supposedly normal elder into one with significant problems. If someone really was well one day and then became cognitively impaired the next day, the cause is likely to be a stroke, not Alzheimer's disease. There are usually other signs pointing to that etiology (e.g., continued neurologic symptoms or signs). Most types of dementia other than stroke occur quite gradually. However, a stroke in someone who already has Alzheimer's disease (which is not uncommon) can cause existing impairment to become significantly worse relatively quickly. It is also common that someone who already has Alzheimer's disease can become suddenly worse cognitively in the face of a relatively minor physical ailment like a urinary tract infection. Fortunately, when the underlying medical problem is appropriately treated, cognition will improve back to baseline, or very close to it, but cognitive improvement can take somewhat longer than physical improvement.

In addition to determining if the symptoms began suddenly or insidiously, the evaluator will want to determine if the decline has continued since the symptoms were first noted. This is the classic pattern in the case of Alzheimer's disease. Individuals who have had cognitive problems for years without further decline probably do not have Alzheimer's disease. Insidious onset and continuing cognitive decline are the clinical hallmarks of the disease.

Activities of Daily Living

In addition to getting a thorough picture of the chief complaint and the pattern of cognitive symptoms, the evaluator determines whether or not instrumental activities of daily living (IADLs; e.g., driving, handling finances, remembering medications) are intact. Individuals who have significant cognitive difficulties but absolutely no impairment in functioning, even in IADLs, may have mild cognitive impairment but probably not Alzheimer's disease. To meet criteria for a diagnosis of Alzheimer's disease, there needs to be some impairment in functioning that affects daily life in some way. Usually, this involves an impairment in IADLs.

The evaluator will also want to determine if basic activities of daily living (ADLs; e.g., dressing, bathing, eating, and toileting) are impaired. While these basic ADLs tend to become impaired only after years of illness and considerable impairment in instrumental activities, it is possible to have a particular difficulty in a single ADL relatively early. Persons who have significant impairment of multiple basic ADLs are likely to need considerable assistance from professional caregivers, if they are to remain out of a nursing home setting. Some tasks such as bathing, changing clothing, and toileting more advanced patients may not be something an older spouse is able to do at home, and adult children may be uncomfortable assisting with these more intimate tasks. It can be a good idea, if it is possible, to have assistance from outside caregivers for many of the basic ADL tasks, so that the spouse or adult children can remain in the role of spouse or child, rather than in the role of nurse.

Mood and Behavioral Symptoms

In addition to assessing cognition and function, the evaluator also determines what if any mood, behavior, or personality changes are part of the current picture. If they are prominent, much of the evaluation may be focused on these concerns (see Chapter 7).

Past History

The evaluator will inquire whether or not the person being examined has ever suffered a significant head injury, particularly with loss of consciousness. Even head injuries many years earlier may be associated with an increased risk of cognitive impairment in the present. The memory specialist will also want to determine if the person had cognitive difficulties at any time in the more remote past, although this is uncommon. Learning about past history also includes inquiring about previous psychiatric difficulties.

Family History

It is important to determine if there are any genetically related family members who have suffered from Alzheimer's disease. In the case of older individuals being evaluated at present, it is likely that if a mother or father suffered from Alzheimer's disease, it may not have been diagnosed as such, but the history of increasing forgetfulness, a nursing home placement, and so forth might give strong clues. People with a direct relative (parent or sibling) with

Alzheimer's disease have an increased risk of developing the disease compared to those who do not have a family history, although this is by no means inevitable. However, if there is a very strong family history, with multiple direct relatives suffering from the disease, this information may influence the treatment decisions by the memory specialist and it may be advisable to follow such a vulnerable individual at more frequent intervals than others without this history.

Personal History

The memory specialist will determine the level of education of the individual being evaluated, as it can influence the outcome of the cognitive examination. Some office-based cognitive examinations do take into account the level of education when determining the significance of a given score on the test. In addition to education, the memory specialist will likely ask about the individual's employment history and whether any cognitive problems on the job led to retirement. A description of current interests, hobbies, and how the individual spends a typical day can be quite illuminating. Also, the evaluator will want to know about community connections such as church, friends, and so forth. There is some evidence that individuals who have a strong network of social support are less likely to develop Alzheimer's disease compared to those who are more isolated. And significant sources of support will certainly have implications for the future for both the afflicted individual and the family.

It is also very important for the evaluator to inquire about children—how many there are, how many live nearby, and the nature of their relationship to the individual being assessed. It is certainly easier for someone with Alzheimer's disease when the Alzheimer's family is large, supportive, and nearby to help with tasks, with caregiving, and with providing companionship for both the person with Alzheimer's disease and the primary caregiver.

Medical History

As discussed in Chapter 2, many medical conditions and medications can have a significant impact on memory, thinking, concentration, and other cognitive functions. A change in medication or treatment of an underlying medical condition may improve if not totally eliminate the cognitive difficulty. If there is a significant history of past or present alcohol use, this must be noted. Ongoing heavy alcohol consumption will need to brought under control before any accurate assessment of cognition can occur. Depression, anxiety, and other psychiatric conditions, especially if untreated, can also cause significant cognitive difficulties, not to mention general distress.

The Mental Status Examination

The evaluating physician will note the individual's appearance, overall level of cooperation, general mood, whether or not there are any psychotic signs or symptoms, and the overall style and facility of the individual's communications. The evaluator will observe the individual's current mood and range of affect and note whether there appears to be any anxiety at the time of the interview.

The Cognitive Examination

Some cognitive testing is generally done during the assessment. Several brief cognitive tests are commonly used for this purpose. They usually take only a few minutes and are generally well tolerated, unless the individual has considerable cognitive problems or defensiveness about his or her difficulties. Ideally, the evaluator performs the cognitive examination in a comfortable atmosphere of inquiry, giving significant positive feedback for all answers that are reasonably correct and making note of, but not emphasizing, those questions that are not correctly answered. Once again, this part of the evaluation should focus on what remains preserved in the individual's abilities, not what is wrong. Many patients find cognitive testing quite traumatic, and an empathic memory specialist may decide to terminate testing for the time being, even if all important information has not been gathered, rather than forcing the patient to do something that is obviously humiliating or otherwise uncomfortable. Generally, no one who is cognitively normal objects to cognitive testing; only those with cognitive problems will complain or become anxious or tense when the cognitive examination is being administered. Even people who score very well but have considerable anxiety or stress while undergoing the test likely have some degree of cognitive impairment. This is one reason why it is important for evaluators to perform cognitive testing themselves rather than simply relying on a test result handed to them by the office staff; it is critical to observe how the person undertakes this critical task, rather than simply reviewing the results of a test performed by someone else.

The Physical Examination

As part of the evaluation, a physical examination may be performed if it has not been done very recently; certain areas of the physical or neurologic examination may be repeated to ensure that certain conditions are not present that could be contributing to the current cognitive symptoms.

Blood Tests

Several blood tests are typically performed as part of a thorough cognitive evaluation, to rule out unexpected but generally readily treatable causes of cognitive difficulties. The following laboratory tests are most commonly recommended:

- Complete blood count
- Blood glucose
- Kidney function tests
- Liver function tests
- Vitamin B_{12} levels
- Thyroid screening

Depending on the medical history, the physician may also want to obtain other laboratory tests. Occasionally this will include an analysis of cerebrospinal fluid to ensure there is no infection in the brain.

Genetic Testing

Genetic testing, generally for the APO E allele pattern, is usually not performed, unless as part of a research battery. See Chapter 2 for a discussion of the role of APO E in Alzheimer's disease.

Head Imaging

Head imaging (CT, MRI, or PET scan of the brain) is commonly but not universally performed as part of the diagnostic assessment. No head imaging study in common use is able to make a positive diagnosis of Alzheimer's disease or any of the other common dementias, but can be very helpful in ruling out the presence of a brain tumor, stroke, blood clot, or other lesion that could cause or contribute to the symptoms. A diagnosis of vascular dementia almost always requires head imaging evidence of small or large strokes or other vascular damage in the brain, in addition to cognitive symptoms.

Neuropsychological Testing

A more extensive battery of neuropsychological testing can be useful in delineating more precisely the areas of cognitive difficulty or obtaining a detailed measure of current cognitive abilities to compare to a previous or future point. One would want to weigh the importance of obtaining this information, over and above the information gathered in the careful interview and brief mental status test, considering the stress (and cost) of a lengthy battery for someone with cognitive impairments. The clinician can often be helpful in making decisions as to whether or not such testing is necessary.

RESULTS OF THE DIAGNOSTIC EVALUATION

Following the diagnostic evaluation—either at the time of the initial assessment or on a follow-up visit scheduled after further testing such as MRI, blood tests, and possibly neuropsychological testing—the memory specialist will generally share his or her diagnostic impressions and recommendations. Different memory specialists have different practices in this regard, but generally it is best if the person who has been evaluated and the accompanying family members are given as specific a diagnosis as possible. If a decision is made not to tell the person being evaluated that he or she has Alzheimer's disease, there should be a clear and positive reason why it is being withheld, beyond the general discomfort of the subject. Many family members assume that their loved one would somehow be harmed by being told the diagnosis. While this fear is understandable, most studies show that this is not the case. In general, families manage this difficult situation much better when no secrets are kept from the person with the disease. The clinician should encourage the family to give as much information as possible to the person with memory difficulties. This may be another situation where some stretching of the truth may be warranted, in order not to leave the person with the disease feeling hopeless. For example, it may be useful to say that the evaluation suggested that the individual may have "a mild case" of Alzheimer's disease, even if there is significant impairment. It can be helpful to add that it is certainly good that it was diagnosed at this time, rather than later, as getting started sooner rather than later with treatment can make an important difference. If the afflicted individual has an older sibling or a parent who had Alzheimer's, it may be important to stress that the ability to treat the disease has advanced considerably in recent years, and outcomes witnessed with a parent or older sibling are not necessarily inevitable in the present situation.

The memory specialist who has made the diagnosis may not see the individual (and the family) again at all, or will see them only infrequently. It is therefore especially important that the clinician working with a family member who has just been diagnosed with Alzheimer's disease be available regularly to the family for support and to answer some of the many questions that will inevitably arise. And it is critical for clinicians to indicate that they will be working hard with the family to do all that can be done to lessen the impact of the disease and ensure that a good quality of life continues as long as possible.

At times, the results of an initial evaluation are inconclusive, and no firm diagnosis can be made. This commonly occurs when an individual appears to have mild cognitive impairment but no definite signs of dementia. It is important to make clear what is known while stressing that the outcome of this condition is quite uncertain. It is possible that the person will revert to normal, continue to have mild cognitive impairment for some time, or progress to Alzheimer's. The current state of our knowledge does not permit us to make an accurate prediction of the person's future. In uncertain diagnostic situations, the passage of time is the best— and sometimes the only—way to clarify the situation. This situation is anxiety provoking for all, and it is critical that the clinician be readily available to the family for support during this uncertain period.

CHAPTER 4

The Long Journey

Once a diagnosis has been made, the primary caregiver and other members of the Alzheimer's family must recognize and accept the fact that they are facing a long journey and need to prepare for it, practically and emotionally. Although no one can foresee all that will be involved, and therefore cannot fully prepare for what lies ahead, there are a number of imperatives for the Alzheimer's family that will immeasurably help them manage the difficult journey they are now facing.

INITIATE A RELATIONSHIP WITH A CLINICIAN

Busy medical practitioners today are rarely able to answer the myriad questions, provide all the information and support, and offer the therapeutic expertise that the Alzheimer's caregiver and other family members need. They lack the time, and in some cases they lack the specific expertise needed to carefully and successfully guide family members through this long, difficult journey. Indeed, the purpose of this book is to prepare clinicians to become skilled counselors for the Alzheimer's family. Those families who avail themselves of this added expertise will be better equipped to cope with this task, which is often described by caregivers as the most difficult undertaking of their life.

While reading books and going to lectures about Alzheimer's disease is very important (see below), many questions can only be answered by someone who has come to know the family (through the primary caregiver or other family members) and understands its structure and its particular strengths and weakness. Even very sophisticated families are at a loss to know how to begin to care for a loved one with Alzheimer's disease and will have innumerable questions that need to be answered. While the afflicted person's physician should and will address some of these questions, particularly about the illness itself, many will have to do with caregiving and the caregiver, which will likely not be addressed by the physician. The following are examples of some of the important questions family members will ask the clinician:

- How should I respond when she says she doesn't want to do something I think she should do?
- Should I try to get him to remember something, or should I just supply the information?
- How do we address the issue of her driving?
- Is it a good idea for him to travel to Florida with my granddaughter?
- Why am I feeling so angry all the time?

Family members who work closely with a clinician throughout the course of a loved one's illness are better able to cope with the challenges that arise and are less stressed in the process.

ANTICIPATORY GRIEF AND AMBIGUOUS LOSS

Anticipatory grief refers to the grief one feels when a death or other loss is expected but hasn't yet occurred. Anticipatory grief may be a more difficult emotion than pure grief; in anticipatory grief, the loved one is both present and not present at the same time. One cannot really "move on" as is necessary in resolving grief, when there is still so much caregiving to do.

Another useful concept related to anticipatory grief is *ambigu-*

ous loss (Boss, 1999), which refers to the discordant feeling that comes from interacting with a person with Alzheimer's who is physically alive but no longer seems present socially or psychologically. As with anticipatory grief, ambiguous loss is difficult for individuals to come to grips with on their own.

Caregivers have indicated that the gradual loss of their loved one to the disease, along with the pain of letting go, are the most difficult aspects of being an Alzheimer's caregiver. The clinician can play a critical role in helping to elucidate and work through these difficult emotions of anticipatory grief and ambiguous loss. Family members will manage best when they face these issues squarely, without denial and avoidance. The family is witnessing the slow death of their loved one, and there is nothing they or anyone else can do to prevent that from happening. Although most family members try to maintain a sense of cheerfulness with the afflicted person, and do not like to talk about the fatal nature of Alzheimer's disease, that painful reality needs to be faced by the caregiver, nevertheless. Encouraging family members to review the various losses that have occurred and will occur as the disease progresses and helping family members to experience this grief fully is one of the most valuable tasks a clinician can undertake.

Many caregivers harbor feelings that they wish the person with Alzheimer's disease would simply die, and invariably they feel very guilty about having such thoughts. It can be very helpful for the clinician to normalize these feelings, pointing out that these emotions and sentiments are indeed very common in this situation. It can be quite helpful for the clinician to simply listen to the caregiver's expressions of grief, without trying to make the person feel better and certainly without conveying the idea that it's not that bad; it *is* that bad, and worse. It is common for the family member to express a great deal of gratitude to the clinician for the opportunity to vent these painful feelings so openly. It is pleasing to see how helpful this can be, but it also may make clear how little the caregiver is sharing these feelings with anyone else. It would be useful for the clinician to suggest that the caregiver try to discuss these painful emotions with a close friend or family member, in addition to continuing this useful process with the clinician. It is generally not helpful for caregivers to share the extent of their grief with the afflicted one; even though the person with Alzheimer's was previously the one person with whom the caregiver would discuss serious matters such as these, that is no longer possible now that the illness has developed. Trying to have this discussion with the afflicted individual will only make both feel worse and will add a layer of guilt to the caregiver's already significant burden.

DIFFERENTIATING CAREGIVER SADNESS FROM DEPRESSION

As caregivers allow themselves to experience the grief of their losses, their sadness can be intense and palpable. Some caregivers are able to compartmentalize these feelings and continue functioning reasonably normally. They are sad, to be sure, about their loved one, but at other moments they are able to experience the pleasures of day-to-day life, to enjoy the company of others, and to pursue their own personal interests. Their grief has not turned into a more pervasive state of depression. Others, however, seem to be taken over by the grief and begin to lose the ability to function or to feel a sense of enjoyment in anything they do. In their sadness, they become less effective in their daily life and in the task of caregiving. These caregivers have progressed from simple grief to depression.

It can be quite challenging for the clinician to determine whether the family member is merely grieving or has entered a state of depression. Furthermore, grief and depression may exist on a continuum, with the difference between them being more a matter of degree than a qualitative difference. It is important for the clinician to try to make this important differential diagnosis, however. In doing so, it may help to consider several questions:

- Is there any variability in the caregiver's mood?
- Are there moments of joy, in addition to sadness, or is the individual's mood consistently low?

- Is the caregiver able to function normally in daily activities, including caregiving tasks, or has this ability declined?
- Has the caregiver become noticeably more irritable or guilty, or shown any other significant changes in interactions with the afflicted person or with others?
- Are basic functions like eating and sleeping consistently impaired?

One needs to judge these matters over a period of weeks, rather than a single day or two. Caregivers can have bad days, just like people with Alzheimer's disease. A diagnosis of depression merits at least a consultation with a physician and possibly antidepressant medication. Such medications are not likely to be helpful in simple grief. However, with grief or depression, supportive counseling can be quite beneficial to help improve mood. In addition, someone who has worked through issues of grief earlier in the disease process will be better able to cope with the ongoing distress this illness will cause over time.

GET AS MUCH INFORMATION AND EDUCATION ABOUT ALZHEIMER'S DISEASE AS POSSIBLE

One of the best tools for managing Alzheimer's disease is to learn as much as possible about it. Many excellent books have been written for the caregiver about Alzheimer's disease, which can be purchased or obtained in many town libraries (see Readings and Resources). In addition, many videos are now available for people who prefer to learn that way, and there is ample information about Alzheimer's disease online (see Readings and Resources for a list of some of the best sites). With so much information available, there really is no reason for a family member not to learn a great deal about the illness. The investment of time to learn is always worthwhile. Some family members will indicate that they do not want to spend time reading about the disease—that when they have time available, they would rather focus on something other than Alzheimer's. That sentiment is certainly understandable, but in the long run, people who have learned as much as they can about the illness will handle it better and will have more time to themselves as a result.

In many communities, there are periodic presentations on Alzheimer's disease, through a senior center, a local college, nursing care facility, or hospital. In addition, the Alzheimer's Association, which has chapters in nearly every community in the country, regularly offers a number of programs for family members and other caregivers. These free programs may feature local experts or staff from the Alzheimer's Association. Information about the local chapter and its schedule of educational programs can be found on the national Alzheimer's Association Web site (www.alz.org).

Learning about Alzheimer's disease involves continuing education; the person with the disease changes continuously, so areas that were of concern in the past may not be relevant now, while new issues have developed. Also, there are new developments in the field on a regular basis, and attending good educational programs should help keep the family member up to date.

Finally, knowledge of the disease will also create a sense of some control over it. Being able to feel some control—or, perhaps more accurately, not to feel out of control—in the face of this illness is one of the most important ways to modulate the enormous stress associated with being a caregiver. With Alzheimer's caregiving, knowledge is power.

ATTEND AN ALZHEIMER'S SUPPORT GROUP ON A REGULAR BASIS

Alzheimer's support groups exist in most communities. Local newspapers usually list them, or they can be found on the Alzheimer's Association's Web site. Attending a support group is an excellent way to learn about the disease and, especially, about ways to cope with it. A support group also offers family members an opportunity to talk about their particular situation and their emotional reactions in a setting where others are not judgmental and family members can feel that they are not alone. Support groups are anonymous (there are no records of who attends, and members are instructed not to discuss the meetings with others) and there are no charges. Many groups also include educational sessions as part of their regular schedule.

In spite of how valuable they can be, only a small minority of caregivers and family members attend support groups, unfortunately. Most feel that they are not able to spend the required amount of time away from the person with Alzheimer's disease; or they feel that the group is at an inconvenient time or place; or they feel that they don't really need the group or don't generally benefit from this type of activity. All of these may be rationalizations, covering over the anxiety the caregiver feels about attending and sharing experiences and feelings. Another reason people avoid support groups is that they fear hearing about other situations that seem even worse. However, this form of denial, while understandable, is not in the caregiver's best interest. Knowing what lies ahead, although it may be very sad or frightening, helps the family member prepare, emotionally and practically, for the future.

The clinician should strongly encourage the family member to attend a support group, exploring the various rationalizations that are offered to avoid it. Family members who resist the idea of going can be asked to make a commitment to at least attend one support group meeting. If they do, many people will want to continue, because they find the atmosphere unexpectedly comforting and positive. Caregivers and other family members both benefit from the opportunity to vent about their situation with others who understand, and they can learn valuable caregiving tips from others who have been through very similar circumstances.

DIVIDE CAREGIVING TASKS AMONG ALL FAMILY MEMBERS (NEAR AND FAR)

All caregivers become stressed by the burdens of caring for someone with Alzheimer's disease, but to the extent that those burdens are shared with other members of the family, the stress is usually reduced and is more manageable. However, the division of caregiving tasks among the various members of the Alzheimer's family is often very unequal. It is natural to have one primary caregiver, but there is no reason why that person must do everything, if other family members are in the vicinity. Certainly, some caregivers do not feel that any other members of the Alzheimer's family could do the job properly; these primary caregivers complain that no one helps, but they may be quite reluctant to accept help from others in the first place. Other family members may sense the proprietary attitude of the caregiver toward the person with dementia and stay away as a result. It may also be that the primary caregiver's attitude is convenient for other members of the family, since they want the best for their loved one but don't necessarily want their own life significantly inconvenienced to make sure that happens.

Living spouses usually take on the majority of the caregiving tasks (assuming they are physically and cognitively well enough to do it). Frequently, well spouses feel that the responsibility of caring for the afflicted spouse is theirs, alone, and do not wish to burden the adult children with it. However, in the long run (and this journey is, indeed, a long run), it is best that the tasks of caregiving be shared as much as possible among all of the members of the Alzheimer's family who live nearby. Other tasks can and should be assigned to adult children who live some distance away, if at all possible. Adult children who live far away might contribute financially. Even if it is a small amount, it will help not only with the enormous costs of the disease but with the sense of sharing the burden among all family members. The job of caring for someone with Alzheimer's disease is simply too much for anyone to undertake alone. And there will be less intrafamily tension if the responsibility is viewed as a shared one from the beginning.

Soon after the diagnosis, there should be a meeting of all family members. If there is a living nondemented spouse, it is appropriate for him or her to be officially in charge, although assigning various caregiving tasks to different members of the family should be a cooperative effort among all. It is best if each individual selects those tasks which suit his or her interests and abilities. One person might be in charge of making sure medications are properly taken; another might be responsible for any home repairs or outside maintenance that becomes necessary; a third might be the liaison with health care providers, going to all doctors' appointments, and so forth. All of the available family members need to be assigned times to provide supervision for the afflicted parent, even if one of the children lives with the parent. While that individual may provide a greater share of the supervision, others need to step in regularly to allow the person who lives with the afflicted individual to have times off duty.

The clinician can play an important role in helping the family divide up tasks in this fashion. It would be very useful for the clinician to meet with as many family members as possible, as a group, as early in the illness as possible, to emphasize the importance of dividing up the tasks in an equitable way and helping with the negotiations to establish them. Follow-up meetings may well be necessary, particularly if members of the family are not following through on their commitments, or as the situation changes and new tasks are needed to be performed by others.

ENSURE THAT THE PRIMARY CAREGIVER HAS REGULAR PERIODS OF RESPITE

Periods of respite for the primary caregiver are critical. Almost nothing works as well to relieve the stress of caregiving as having regular periods of time when one is completely free of the responsibility. Everyone, even those who dearly love their jobs, needs regular time off—weekends, evenings, vacations, and so forth. The same is true for the person who has the job of primary caregiver. No matter how devoted a spouse might be to the person with Alzheimer's disease, it is essential to have regular periods when that person is not caregiving. It is critical that respite periods come on a regular basis, so that when people are back on duty they already know when their next day, or afternoon, or weekend off will be. And it is only respite when the individual is not only not providing care but is able to relax knowing that some other reliable person is in charge. Respite is not a run to the mall for a couple of hours, calling home regularly and worrying the whole time about the afflicted person who has been left home alone. That type of situation increases, not decreases, stress.

Depending on the type and intensity of needs of the person with Alzheimer's, the nature of the relationship between the afflicted person and the primary caregiver, and the degree of burden the primary caregiver experiences, respite periods may be shorter or longer, less frequent or more frequent. They need to be often enough and long enough so that the primary caregiver feels replenished by them, but this varies so much that it is impossible to prescribe a frequency or duration in the abstract. Clinicians can make specific suggestions about respite depending on their understanding of the situation.

What the family member does with respite time is also quite variable, but ideally should include activities that have nothing to do with the person with Alzheimer's disease or the management of the household. It should be something the caregiver would define as fun, perhaps going out to dinner and a movie with a good friend, going shopping with an adult daughter, going on a weekend foliage tour with a fraternal organization, or simply sitting and reading a book. Many spousal caregivers prefer to spend at least some of their respite times relaxing in their own home. If that is the case, the person with Alzheimer's needs to be taken out somewhere for that period of time, because few primary caregivers can truly feel they are off duty if their afflicted loved one is just downstairs or in another room.

It can be difficult to get spouses to agree to have periods of respite. Wives, in particular, may simply state that they have not had any interests outside the marital relationship for decades or participated in any independent activities at all during their marriage. That may certainly be true, but the clinician should point out that the marital relationship was not based on caregiving over all of these years, as it is now. It is the caregiving from which they need a break periodically. The clinician should strongly encourage these spouses (or occasionally adult children or others) to develop an interest outside of the home—whether it be cultivating an old friendship, volunteering at the local library, taking an adult education course, or a small part-time job in a local business. This will be helpful now and invaluable once the caregiver is widowed (this topic is discussed in greater detail in Chapter 10).

An excellent way for the primary caregiver and other family members to have regular periods of respite and to benefit the person with Alzheimer's disease at the same time is to enroll him or her in an adult day program. These programs are perhaps best used somewhat later in the disease process, rather than the earliest stages of the illness. Adult day programs can be found in many but not all areas. Some are able to provide transportation to and from home. In many cases, the primary caregiver or other member of the Alzheimer's family will need to transport the person back and forth. Adult day programs offer an opportunity for socialization and structured activities. They give the person a valuable change of environment. Importantly, they provide the primary caregiver an opportunity to be free of caregiving responsibilities for a period of time, to go to work, do errands, pursue other interests, or simply have some time off from the burdens of caregiving, while knowing that the person with Alzheimer's is in a safe and therapeutic setting. This is invaluable in helping caregivers manage the stress of caregiving.

Many people with Alzheimer's disease will resist going, as they are more comfortable staying in familiar surroundings at home, and they prefer being with their spouse over being with anyone else. Yet it is extremely important to help the person with Alzheimer's become comfortable being cared for by someone other than the primary caregiver. It may take several attempts to engage the person in such a program; the caregiver may need to be very forceful about the need for the person with Alzheimer's to do it for both of them, or it may not happen at all, because of resistance that makes the fighting or the guilt too great to bear. Families who regularly utilize an adult day program usually feel it is tremendously valuable to them to have the respite time, and those with Alzheimer's disease who ultimately agree to attend frequently enjoy the program immensely and look forward to going as often as possible. However, too often family members will utilize the program for only a few hours at a time, not long enough for the person with Alzheimer's to feel connected, and not long enough for the caregiver to benefit sufficiently. Limited use of these programs often appears to be a compromise because of guilt—at least initially because the individual does not want to go, and because the caregiver does not really feel entitled to the break. The clinician should examine these attitudes and try to help the family member modify them, so that the adult day program or similar activities can be optimally utilized.

CHAPTER 5

Maintaining a Connection

In Chapter 4, the need to begin to grieve the loss of the person with Alzheimer's disease was emphasized. Indeed, grieving is a continuous process throughout the course of the illness; new losses occur on a regular basis, and the Alzheimer's family must continuously adapt to the changing, and diminishing, person. Yet at the same time, most people with Alzheimer's disease live for many years following the diagnosis, and thus the family, in spite of its grieving, must also cope with the challenge of maintaining a relationship with the afflicted person, in the face of growing impairment. These seemingly opposite tasks—grieving and working to maintain a connection—make each other more challenging for the Alzheimer's family. Yet both of them are vital both for the individual with the disease and for the members of the Alzheimer's family.

This chapter addresses two different areas that involve maintaining a sense of connection to the loved one with Alzheimer's: (1) coping with communication challenges; and (2) finding appropriate activities to pursue in the face of growing cognitive and functional difficulties, including physically intimate activities with the afflicted spouse.

COPING WITH COMMUNICATION CHALLENGES

In Chapter 2, it was noted that aphasia—language impairment—is one of the cardinal features of Alzheimer's disease. This involves expressive language (i.e., the ability of the afflicted individual to express thoughts, feelings, or other information) as well as receptive language (the ability to comprehend language, verbal or written, that is received). The time of onset and severity of this symptom varies, but it is almost always present to a greater or lesser degree relatively early in the disease process and worsens as the disease progresses, to the point when, by the late-moderate or early-severe stage of illness, verbal communication is almost always extremely disordered, limited, or nonexistent.

It is important to remember that, as this happens, the individual does not lose the ability to understand nonverbal language; if anything, the sensitivity to nonverbal communication seems heightened, at least initially, while verbal language skills are deteriorating.

It is also important to keep in mind that, while receptive communication is definitely impaired along with expressive communication in most people with Alzheimer's, receiving and understanding communication is usually better preserved than producing (expressing) communication, at least until late in the disease. Thus, the person who has great difficulty speaking may be able to understand much of what is being said to or around him or her. Too often people talk about someone with Alzheimer's disease as if the individual is not present, even when he is not only present but understands much of what is being said.

In addition to the difficulties with expressive and receptive language, persons with Alzheimer's, of course, have progressive difficulty with short-term memory. As the disease progresses, the ability to hold something in mind for more than a few moments diminishes significantly, so that people with Alzheimer's may begin a sentence and, halfway through, actually forget what they were talking about. They may also be unable to understand longer sentences, paragraphs, or communications that contain multiple ideas, concepts, directions, or facts, for the same reason.

With these considerations in mind, the following is a list of of dos and don'ts for communicating with someone with Alzheimer's disease, which the clinician should consider sharing with the family.

DO

1. Do use techniques to attract and maintain the person's attention. Turn off the television or radio or go to a quiet room and close the door if necessary. Make and maintain eye contact. Place yourself at the same level as the person with Alzheimer's disease. If the afflicted person is sitting, sit down nearby so that your heads are at approximately the same height. Use gestures and touch to facilitate communication and to maintain the attention of the person with Alzheimer's disease.

2. Do make all communications short, simple, and clear. Give only one direction at a time; ask one question; convey only one idea, concept, or piece of information per sentence; and then check to see if it was understood.

3. Do identify yourself to the person with Alzheimer's disease if there is any doubt that he or she knows who you are. While this may not apply to immediate members of the Alzheimer's family until late in the disease, it may apply to more distant family members, even relatively early in the illness. It is better to have someone say, "I know who you are, of course" (even if they don't) than for the person with Alzheimer's to be asked to interact with someone whose identity is unclear. Not only is a name helpful, but offering some additional identifying data may be a good idea, as well. For example, saying, "I'm your nephew Carl, your brother Fred's son" can be quite helpful. It is common that persons with dementia may not recall who someone is, but even if the patient understands that the visitor is a member of the family, he or she may not understand how they are related, and the generations, in particular, can become very confused. Sons are seen as brothers, sisters as aunts, and so forth. It is probably better to err in the direction of identifying oneself. People with Alzheimer's will usually try to act like they know who someone is, when they sense that they are expected to know the individual. It can be confusing for all concerned and it is stressful for the person who is afflicted.

4. Do call the person by name. This helps not only to get and maintain the individual's attention; it also emphasizes that she is the one being addressed. While that may seem obvious to the speaker, it may not be obvious to the person with Alzheimer's disease, even if no one else is in the room. Calling the person by name is also a way to show respect. Use the last name with Mr. or Mrs., rather than the first name, if that is how you would address a similar person who did not have dementia.

5. Do speak slowly. The person with dementia may take longer to accurately process and understand what is being said. Rapid-fire speech may be overwhelming to the afflicted person. Rather than picking up bits and pieces of what was said, the entire communication becomes incomprehensible.

6. Do use closed-ended questions that can be answered "yes" or "no." For example, ask, "Did you enjoy the roast beef and potatoes at dinner?" rather than, "What did you have for dinner?" The latter is experienced as a memory test and probably will not be effective, whereas, "Did you enjoy the roast beef and potatoes" reminds the individual and invites a simple yes or no answer, which is much easier for the afflicted person.

It does no good to try to force individuals to remember something that is not readily available to them, although some people seem to feel this is a good brain exercise for people with Alzheimer's. Mostly, it is an exercise in frustration for them.

7. Do find a different way to say the same thing if it wasn't understood the first time. Usually, a simpler, more concrete statement with fewer words will be better understood. It is important to read the face and reactions of people with Alzheimer's while speaking with them. Do they appear to paying attention? Are their eyes glazing over? Do they become restless and unsettled while being addressed? It may not be completely reliable to simply ask people with Alzheimer's if they understood something, as they will almost always answer positively whether or not they actually did. In addition, it can be demeaning to them, whether or not the communication was comprehended. A better technique to be certain that a message is understood is to ask the individual to repeat it back, "just to make sure it was clear." This seems less like a test of the memory of the person with Alzheimer's, and more like a test for the speaker, which is certainly better.

8. Do use distraction, partial truths, or even fiblets when necessary, if telling the whole truth will upset the person with dementia. For example, in answer to the question, "Where is my mother?" it might be better to say "She's not here right now" rather than "She died 20 years ago."

Very understandably, many people have trouble with this approach. They have never told a lie to their mother or spouse and find it very difficult to do so now. For those who cannot bring themselves to be dishonest, simply avoiding and changing the subject as fast as possible may be the best approach, although that is sometimes not successful. While honesty is generally the correct way to handle all interactions, there are times when situational ethics seem to apply. What is the overall goal at this point? Taking into account someone's illness, the most important goal may well be to avoid unnecessary stress or distress for the patient, if at all possible. Some would feel that a small untruth, or partial truth— "She's not here right now"—is ethically acceptable; the end (avoiding stress and distress in the person with Alzheimer's) justifies the means. These little lies or partial truths have been called fiblets"—little fibs that are acceptable in the larger context.

9. Do use repetition as much as necessary. Be prepared to say the same things over and over because the person with dementia cannot recall them for more than a few moments at a time.

One of the more frequent features of living with someone with Alzheimer's, and a common source of stress, is repetitiveness. People with Alzheimer's will ask the same question, over and over, because they cannot remember having asked it before, or cannot remember the answer, or both. This seems to occur with greater intensity when the subject of the question is one that causes some anxiety. It may be that anxiety over who is coming for dinner tonight may cause the forgetting to happen even more rapidly.

Repetitiveness is a core feature of Alzheimer's disease, but when it intensifies, it might be helpful for a family member to say something reassuring, such as, "The Smiths are coming. They are our old friends and they only plan to stay a short while." It is a rare caregiver who never gets somewhat annoyed after being asked the same question a dozen times in the course of an hour or two. It is necessary for the caregiver to understand the reasons for the repetitiveness—it is caused by the impairment in recent memory, which is a core symptom of Alzheimer's disease. The individual is not doing it on purpose; most of the time people with Alzheimer's are completely unaware that they are being repetitive, although occasionally they will have an awareness that they have asked the same question before but cannot recall the answer.

Sometimes it is helpful to write down the answer to the frequently repeated question and have the person keep it. The statement "The Smiths are coming at 6 o'clock" with a drawing of a clock, the hands pointing to 6, might be useful for some. However, other afflicted individuals may not be able to remember to look at the paper, or to realize that it applies to the question they have been repetitively asking.

10. Do be aware that the tone in which something is said may be as important as the actual content. As discussed above, although people with Alzheimer's disease frequently lose the ability to comprehend speech, they generally maintain a keen ability to read nonverbal communication, including body language, facial expressions, and tone of voice. The ability to read and respond to these nonverbal elements of communication is greatest, of course, with members of the Alzheimer's family. Even late in the disease, the person with Alzheimer's seems quite aware of whether family members smile, and whether they speak in a soothing, calm, pleasant tone, or an impatient, irritated one, even if they understand nothing of the content. It is critical for the family members to be very aware of the importance of these aspects of communication, which convey emotions more than ideas or other content.

DON'T

1. Don't ever say the following:

- "Do you remember?"
- "Did you forget . . . ?"

- "How could you not know that?"
- "Try to remember!"

It does not help the situation to make this type of remark to the afflicted person who has forgotten something. These comments often are made as a way for the family member to express frustration or anger about the forgetting. While that may be very understandable, it is destructive in that it can only serve to make the person with Alzheimer's feel worse about the deficit.

The final statement, "Try to remember!" is futile. Once something is forgotten, no amount of effort is likely to bring it back. Certainly the pressure created by such a comment will make someone less likely, not more likely, to recall whatever was forgotten.

2. Don't ask questions that directly challenge short-term memory. Don't say, "Do you remember what we did last night?" The honest answer will likely be "no," and this may be humiliating for people with dementia, after they try unsuccessfully to guess the answer. Similarly, rather than saying, "Do you remember me?," the well-meaning family member visiting from out of town is better off saying, "I'm your nephew Carl, your brother Fred's son," as mentioned above.

3. Don't talk in paragraphs. People with Alzheimer's disease are often unable to follow a complex set of ideas. It is best to present just one idea at a time; one noun and one verb in each sentence is usually enough. After giving this information, the speaker should pause, allowing time for processing and possibly checking to see if the ideas were understood before continuing.

4. Don't say anything that points out the person's memory difficulty. Avoid remarks like, "I just told you that" or "We already talked about that"—just repeat what you said again (and again). Exasperated family members will make this type of comment as a way of expressing their frustration; of course, it is not at all helpful to people with Alzheimer's and only increases their sense of incompetency.

5. Don't talk in front of the person as if he were not present. Always include the person with dementia in any conversation when he is physically present. As noted above, afflicted individuals may comprehend much more than is apparent and more than they are able to express. Whether or not the words are understood, though, the emotional tone of the conversation is likely to be. Equally importantly, talking about someone who is present as if she is not in the room is demeaning and further reduces the individual's sense of self. Even if there is little chance that much is being understood, it is important to try to include the afflicted individual in any conversation. Making eye contact with the person with Alzheimer's, even while talking with a third person, shows respect. And periodic comments to the afflicted person, such as "How does that sound to you?" can help him feel like part of the conversation.

6. **Don't use lots of pronouns.** In a sentence such as, "Mary went to meet her sister at the train, but when she got there, she had already left," it can be unclear who did what. "Mary went to meet her sister Susan at the train, but when Mary got there, Susan had already left" is better, even if the meaning would be clear the first way to someone not demented.

7. **Don't use slang, unfamiliar words, or jargon.** The latest expressions in common parlance may not be understood by the person with dementia. "We will have dinner every night at six going forward" is more confusing than "After tonight, we will have dinner at six every night." Similarly, expressions like "at the end of the day" or "the rollout will be next week" should be avoided unless they refer to a specific time in the day, or something that is actually on wheels.

8. **Don't use patronizing language or baby talk.** Even very demented persons are sensitive to being talked down to or patronized, and will feel offended, angry, or hurt.

9. **Don't use sarcasm, irony, or similar forms of banter.** This kind of humor can easily backfire and cause hurt or confusion. Although family members may have only the best intentions, attempts at sarcasm or other biting forms of humor can easily be misunderstood and can cause people with Alzheimer's to feel that they are the butt of the joke. A family member who enjoys this

form of banter should practice it with someone other than the afflicted member.

10. Don't be impatient. If you ask a question, wait for a response. Give the person plenty of time to process your question and formulate a response. Trying to speed up the person with Alzheimer's disease is almost never successful, whether in conversation or in almost any other activity.

REMAINING ACTIVE

One of the greatest challenges for the Alzheimer's family is to find activities that they can encourage the afflicted person to pursue, and that they can pursue together to maintain a sense of connection and pleasurable sharing despite the progressive decline that can create a growing chasm between people with Alzheimer's and their loved ones. This need for continued pleasurable sharing certainly includes the need for continuing some form of physical intimacy or sexuality, which almost always changes significantly (see below).

Countering Apathy

The emphasis on activities is important for a number of reasons. Even people with mild Alzheimer's disease frequently have enormous apathy. It is one of the most common and often one of the earliest symptoms of the disease, occurring even before significant memory impairments. Apathy is caused by deterioration in frontal-subcortical circuitry in the brain. The typical signs of apathy are as follows:

- Diminished motivation
- Lack of goal-directed activity
- Loss of interest and goals
- Diminished emotional responsiveness (emotional blunting)

Because of their apathy, people with Alzheimer's disease frequently seem quite content doing very little: sitting in front of the TV without paying much attention to it, looking out the window, or napping off and on throughout the day. This occurs even in persons who have been extremely active their entire lives, prior to the onset of the disease. While it does not particularly bother the person with Alzheimer's to be this way (they are apathetic about it), it is frequently extremely distressing to family members, who often view this as simple laziness or depression. It can be quite valuable for the clinician to help family members understand the concept of apathy and how central it is in Alzheimer's disease. Once the signs of apathy are explained, many family members will immediately recognize that this is precisely what they have been observing and trying to deal with in their loved one.

The other reason for inactivity, of course, is that many of the pursuits the individual used to enjoy may be no longer possible because they are too challenging cognitively. This can apply to activities like playing chess, reading a book, or working on a craft that requires more than repetitive motor activity. It can also apply to socializing with casual friends: Thinking about making conversation, following the conversation of others, remembering the details of people's lives, and talking about oneself are sufficiently stressful that people with Alzheimer's may prefer to avoid these and many other activities.

If individuals afflicted with Alzheimer's appear to be content with very little activity, is this a problem? Shouldn't they simply be left to their own devices? There are times when inactivity is perfectly acceptable; no one with Alzheimer's disease, even those few who do not have apathy, engages in as much activity as they once did—nor should they, probably. Everyone with this disease seems to need periods of quietude during the day or else can become overstimulated, exhausted, and prone to catastrophic reactions (see Chapter 6). In some ways, it may be easier for the Alzheimer's family to care for someone who is content with just sitting; as long as they are present, providing passive caregiving, family members can pursue other activities during these times.

However, there are problems with too much passivity. People with the disease who engage in very little activity may not be discontented, but it would be hard to say they are very happy, either. Mostly, they are just existing, passing time in this state while the disease gets steadily worse. Quality of life may not be terrible, but it is not very positive, either, if one considers quality of life as not only the absence of pain but also the presence of pleasure. There is no firm evidence that the disease progresses more rapidly in those who are apathetic and have very little stimulation compared to those who are not, but such an assumption seems plausible. People with Alzheimer's who pursue a variety of activities that are pleasurable, engage the mind, and involve enjoyable interactions with others appear to maintain the ability to perform a variety of complex tasks, to converse appropriately, and to interact in socially appropriate ways with others longer than those who do not do these things. Whether or not this type of lifestyle affects the rate of disease progression, it may help individuals make the most of the abilities that remain.

Finally, another very important reason to encourage activity is for the sake of the spouse and other family members. The spouse's quality of life will be better if he or she continues to have a partner with whom to engage in various pursuits. That might be as little as an occasional walk around the block, or it might be playing a game of cards, going out for lunch or to a movie, or some other activity on a regular basis. As important as it is for the spouse to maintain connections with other people, independently, one of the great losses for the spouse of someone with Alzheimer's is the gradual loss of a primary companion and partner in a great many different activities. Finally, continuing to include the afflicted family member in the daily life of the family, rather than gradually excluding him or her, helps to maintain that individual's sense of personhood.

How can the Alzheimer's family motivate the apathetic person to engage in activities? Encouragement, cajoling, bargaining, even pleading are all utilized, with varying but usually limited degrees of effectiveness. Asking the individual, "Do it for me" may not be effective because the individual is not able to feel as concerned about the needs or desires of another as he once was. This lack of empathy for the feelings of others occurs even in those who had previously been very thoughtful. Saying that the activities are "doctor's orders" might sometimes be a useful directive, if the afflicted individual seems like someone who would be concerned about that. However, in the end, it can be extraordinarily difficult to engage someone who has significant apathy. Having an attitude that engagement is expected and creating an environment that somehow does not allow the person to exclude himself from family life may help in some ways, along with sometimes simply insisting that the person do something. It may be useful for the clinician to encourage families to take a very firm, insistent stance and only drop this if it creates a great deal of tension or hard feelings. Many family members will not be very insistent because it makes them too angry, or hurt, to be rebuffed; or they may not be insistent because they are not completely convinced of the importance of keeping their loved one engaged. Some, unfortunately, no longer enjoy the company of their family member and would prefer to do things alone, or with others.

Finding Appropriate Activities

What are the best activities for someone with Alzheimer's disease? The simplest answer is that doing anything is usually better than doing nothing. Activities should generally be enjoyable, although some may be more mundane than others. In fact, turning mundane chores into activities can be a very useful approach. For example, a chore such as unloading the dishwasher and putting away the dishes can easily be turned into an activity; the person with the disease and the family member can do this together, one taking the dishes out of the machine while the other puts away. Guessing where a particular item goes can become part of the activity, since this frequently becomes a challenge for the afflicted individual. This approach emphasizes that activities are not simply the things a person does after finishing all of the daily routines and chores; but some of those daily routines or chores can become activities. Such an approach takes some creativity on the part of the family member, but doing so has clear benefits for both. The act of doing the task, rather than simply getting it done, is what is critical.

Other activities, aside from the daily routines described above, need to be carefully chosen. Perhaps the most important criterion is simply that it be something the person with Alzheimer's enjoys—even if she initially says she doesn't want to do it, because of apathy. Beyond that, activities should have the right fit—not too difficult for the person's cognitive level, but certainly not childish or infantilizing, either. They should be consistent with the individual's past interests. Ideally, activities should engage the mind, although activities that require new learning are not likely to succeed. Activities that provide a sense of mastery or usefulness are essential, since so many people with Alzheimer's disease tend to have low self-esteem and feel that they are of little use to themselves or to others (even though they may not acknowledge feeling this way or even recognize it consciously).

As the disease progresses, noncognitive activities are best. Good activities that do not stress cognition include the following:

- Listening to music
- Enjoying a favorite food
- Going for walks or rides in the car
- Enjoying the visits of young children (in small numbers)
- Pets
- Simple gardening tasks

How many different activities should the person with Alzheimer's have? Not including chores and routines that can be turned into activities by the creative caregiver, the following goals would be reasonable:

1. At least one activity per day that gets the afflicted person out of the house.
2. At least one activity per day that involves interacting with someone outside the family.
3. At least one activity per day that involves some degree of physical movement. This may be no more than a slow walk around the block, assuming physical health permits it.

Ideally, a single activity might involve all of these: going out to the local senior center to participate in an exercise group that also includes some conversation among the participants, for example.

One should not aim to fill the entire day with activities; that is likely to lead to adverse consequences. One well-timed activity—

for example, a car ride late in the day, when restlessness and confusion may be more prominent (see Chapter 6)—can be extremely
valuable.

Occasionally, family members visiting from out of town for a
short while feel that they should create as much activity as possible during the visit. They may get theater tickets, make dinner
plans, drag the afflicted person to the mall, and so forth. This approach to visiting is likely to lead to disappointment, or worse.
This can easily happen over holidays, when many people may
visit the Alzheimer's family home at the same time, and there are
days of nonstop activity in and out of the house. While this may be
something that the person used to enjoy before the illness, it can
be important for the clinician to encourage out-of-town relatives to
keep as close to the current routines as possible during their visit.

Importantly, activities can create opportunities for the primary
caregiver and other members of the Alzheimer's family to engage
in enjoyable quality time with the afflicted member. Listening to
music together, looking at old photo albums, sharing a favorite
snack, or going for a walk may be an opportunity for the spouse to
put aside the demands of being a caregiver for a short while and
focus instead on the relationship with the afflicted person as it
used to be prior to the illness. Creating moments of pleasure in this
way is vital for both and will be remembered by the surviving
spouse long after the person with Alzheimer's dies. Ideally, these
activities should happen every day, as well.

Adult children may find that they now pursue activities with
their mother or father that never occurred prior to the illness.
These moments offer extremely important opportunities for sharing and closeness that can have deep and lasting significance for
the adult child—and presumably for the person with the disease,
as well. These activities can, in fact, help improve or repair a previously difficult relationship with the now-afflicted parent. Having
Alzheimer's may make a parent more approachable than before
the illness. The clinician should strongly encourage adult children
or other family members whose relationship with the person with
Alzheimer's has not been ideal to attempt to reengage on a more
positive note. Many of the deep-seated resentments that may have

been felt on both sides are no longer accessible to the person with Alzheimer's, giving the adult child the opportunity—if he or she can set those feelings aside—to redefine the relationship on more positive terms. Adult children who do not take this opportunity to try to improve their relationship with their parent may always feel guilty that they did not do more, no matter who was originally "at fault" for the troubled relationship. And if they make the effort to improve their relationship, they will likely feel very grateful for the new closeness that develops in the final years of the afflicted parent's life. It would seem that, in addition to the benefits to the person with Alzheimer's, the opportunity to feel better in the long term about a difficult parental relationship is well worth the effort and uncomfortable feelings that reaching out in this way might cause the adult child, although many will not be able to take advantage of this new opportunity without some careful coaching from the clinician.

MAINTAINING PHYSICAL INTIMACY WITH A SPOUSE WITH ALZHEIMER'S DISEASE

Usually, one of the most important communications and pleasurable activities between spouses throughout a marriage is physical intimacy. Maintaining this aspect of a relationship can be quite challenging in the face of progressive Alzheimer's disease, for numerous reasons. It can be very helpful for the clinician to inquire about the sexual life of the couple currently, particularly since spouses may be quite uncomfortable volunteering information about this aspect of the relationship.

Interest in sexual intimacy changes in Alzheimer's disease. Many victims of the disease lose interest in sex as the disease progresses (although for some, the opposite happens). Many medications that are used to treat Alzheimer's can lessen sexual drive or performance abilities. For example, selective serotonin reuptake inhibitors, such as citalopram, sertraline, paroxetine, or fluoxetine, are frequently used for depression, irritability, or anxiety in this population. All of these medications can have a significant negative effect on libido and sexual performance.

Less commonly, some afflicted individuals appear to develop sexual apraxia; that is, they simply no longer seem to know how to perform intimate acts, just as they may no longer remember how to properly use utensils at the dining table. Others may remember how to perform, and do so, but forget it soon afterward and complain to their spouse about their lack of a physical relationship.

For the spouse of the afflicted person, the situation is complex, and multiple factors can be involved. As the spouse's view of the partner changes from an intimate, mutual, physically appealing person to a sick, at times childlike person in need of a significant amount of nurturing care, the desire for sex may well diminish. Well spouses may feel they are having sex with a child rather than an adult partner and may be quite bothered by the implications of that. For many, sexual activity ceases once incontinence develops.

In addition, the well spouse may have developed a significant amount of unresolved anger or resentment as a result of the illness, and this alone can put an end to physical desire for the afflicted partner. Finally, the well partner may feel uncomfortable about engaging in sex with someone who may no longer be able to give meaningful consent or indeed even really know who the spouse is.

In spite of these burdens, it is very important for the couple to maintain a sense of physical closeness, although this may well take a different form than earlier in the relationship. Holding hands, hugging, and massage may replace intercourse or other directly sexual activities. It may be a sacrifice for the well partner to accept that this is the limit of physical intimacy, but for some it may be liberating and bring about a greater level of closeness than before, if sex had become more of an obligatory than a strongly desired part of the relationship.

CHAPTER 6

Safety Issues

One of the most important responsibilities of the Alzheimer's family is to ensure the safety of the individual with the disease. This includes protecting the individual from exploitation; making decisions about if, and for how long, the person with Alzheimer's disease can stay alone in the house without supervision; what is safe for the individual to do at home and what needs to be avoided (e.g., using the stove); when it is no longer safe for the person to live alone; how to address the risk of wandering; and determining when it is no longer safe for the person to drive, either alone or with someone else in the car.

Clearly, there are no absolutely right or wrong answers in any of these matters, except perhaps at the extreme ends of the continuum of illness. Making decisions about safety involves balancing respect for individual freedom and autonomy, on the one hand, versus the maintenance of safety of the individual and others, on the other. Different families make very different decisions in very similar circumstances. Adding to the complexity of the situation is the enormous variability from day to day, and even hour to hour, of persons with dementia. It may be that on many days, a given person with the disease is perfectly safe to be alone, drive, cook, but on bad days is sufficiently more cognitively impaired, so that such activities should not be undertaken. Should someone who is safe to live alone nine days out of ten be forced to give up her independence because of the one day in ten when she is not? Similarly, someone may be perfectly safe to use the stove to make breakfast, but by suppertime is much more likely to neglect to turn off a burner.

Safety issues are often the source of some of the greatest tension in Alzheimer's families, when the family wishes to impose some safety restriction on the afflicted member, who strongly resists the limitation on autonomy. This is one area in which people with Alzheimer's have the most difficulty seeing themselves clearly, probably because it involves sophisticated assessments of personal capabilities, on the one hand, and clear assessment of risks on the other. In other words, accurate safety assessment requires a considerable degree of insight and judgment, higher level frontal lobe tasks that are regularly impaired in Alzheimer's disease, often from the earliest stages of illness. Driving and living alone are usually the areas of greatest conflict.

ADVANCE DIRECTIVES

Advance directives can be viewed as a safety measure, in that they keep strangers from making vital decisions for people with Alzheimer's when they are no longer capable of making those decisions. As such, directives are tremendously important for people with Alzheimer's disease, whose decision-making ability will ultimately be lost due to the ravages of the disease. Therefore, the Durable Power of Attorney for Healthcare and the Durable Power of Attorney for Finances are two legal documents that everyone with Alzheimer's disease should complete, if possible. To complete a durable power of attorney (DPOA) in a legally binding way, individuals need to demonstrate that they understand the meaning of the document and are signing it freely without coercion. In the health care DPOA, the signer designates a particular person (usually a spouse or other family member) to be empowered to make medical decisions should the individual become mentally incapacitated. Without this document, hospitals are obligated to go to every extreme to keep someone alive. That may be appropriate in the case of a young person who has had a serious accident, but for someone who is elderly and may have had a serious stroke or a heart arrhythmia with oxygen deprivation and brain damage, it may not be. Being kept alive on machines, at great expense and perhaps physical pain and distress, only to survive severely impaired cognitively, and with little or no quality of life, is not a choice that most people would make. Most life-threatening illnesses that occur in people with Alzheimer's will leave them significantly more impaired than previously, if they survive.

The DPOA for finances is a similar but separate document. It states that if the signer becomes incapacitated mentally, the designated individual will be empowered to make financial decisions on his or her behalf. Because it is a separate document, people are able to designate either the same or a different person to act on their behalf. It is common for persons with Alzheimer's to designate, for example, one child (usually one who lives nearby) as the health care proxy and a different one as the financial proxy.

In the case of both DPOAs, the law clearly states that the designee is required to act according to what the incapacitated individual—not the designee—would want. Of course, the person selecting someone to become a proxy would choose someone who understood and was generally in accord with his or her own views. The proxy has no power unless and until a physician declares that the person has lost the capacity to make health care or financial decisions. People can have capacity for health care decisions but not for finances, or vice versa; therefore, the two powers of attorney do not have to be enacted at the same time.

Most people in the early stages of Alzheimer's disease maintain their capacity for designating a DPOA for health care or for finances. However, an unexpected turn for the worse could change that situation overnight, so it is imperative not to delay the important task of completing these documents. If no DPOA is in place before the individual loses capacity, it may become necessary for a member of the Alzheimer's family to apply for guardianship. This is a much more complicated, lengthy, and expensive process. If it is determined that the afflicted person lacks capacity to make health care or financial decisions, the judge may declare the person incompetent and appoint a guardian. However, if the power of attorney documents are completed while the individual still has capacity, it is likely that guardianship will never be necessary, unless there are strong disagreements among family members about the care of the afflicted person. The clinician should strongly encourage the family to complete these documents as soon as possible, before it becomes too late. The clinician can also make suggestions about which family members might be assigned these tasks, if need be.

EXPLOITATION

Many people with Alzheimer's disease—including those who never fell for a scam earlier in their lives—will be victimized by unscrupulous individuals who are quite aware that a significant segment of the aged population has diminished judgment. Loss of judgment can be a very early symptom of the disease, and it is not uncommon that an episode of exploitation can be the incident that leads the Alzheimer's family to finally recognize that something is seriously amiss. Quite sizable financial losses are not uncommon among those with Alzheimer's disease who have financial means. Other common scams involve invitations to receive magazine subscriptions, with the promise, "You may already be a winner!" or that one could win millions by simply signing up for these periodicals. Most people are appropriately skeptical of the many solicitations that arrive daily in the mail and by e-mail. It is a curious but concerning fact that many people afflicted with the disease so often lose this skepticism. Once the first check is sent to a particular solicitor, one can expect many more requests from the same or similar organizations. As seniors increasingly use the Internet and e-mail, they are more likely to fall prey to the many solicitations that arrive electronically every day. Those whose judgment has become impaired by Alzheimer's disease are unable, it seems, to simply deposit these solicitations in the trash, as most other people do.

Knowing how frequently these events occur, the Alzheimer's family should assume that the afflicted individual will be solicited in some way and may be unable to avoid falling victim, due to impaired judgment. This may be one reason to enact a DPOA for finances, if the person with Alzheimer's is regularly writing checks or, worse, giving credit card information to individuals or organizations not personally known to the family. It is also a reason why people with Alzheimer's disease probably should not have a credit card, in the first place. To help the person maintain some sense of control, it may be a good idea to have a checking account with very limited funds that are replaced only when needed, and after the responsible family member has reviewed the past month's disbursements. Eventually, the individual will lose the ability to write checks, a common deficit in IADLs that occurs relatively early in the illness, but it is certainly possible for significant exploitation to occur before that point.

Even before the individual loses the ability to write checks, and before the DPOA is enacted, it may be a good idea for the spouse or other close member of the family to have a very frank discussion with the person with Alzheimer's about the risks of exploitation, and ask that the person voluntarily appoint a member of the family to assist with managing the financial affairs. This should be one of the first things to consider doing after the diagnosis. For those who are more reluctant to give up control in this way, the family member could ask permission to at least write the checks, while continuing to have the person with Alzheimer's sign them.

LIVING ALONE

Once it becomes apparent that a family member who lives alone has Alzheimer's disease, the family now must consider whether or not it is still safe for the afflicted individual to live alone. Perhaps the person has been living alone for some time or is recently widowed. When one member of a couple dies, it is not uncommon to discover that the surviving spouse has some significant cognitive difficulties that were not previously known. While it is certainly possible that these have worsened (but probably not developed) since the death of the spouse, it may also be that the deceased spouse (assuming that he or she was reasonably cognitively intact) was covering for the spouse who is now alone. Members of couples do this regularly, not necessarily intentionally trying to hide the other's deficits, but in a more gradual and natural way, taking over more and more of the tasks and decisions, serving more and more as the memory for both, and increasingly shielding the demented spouse from the outside world, including even members of the family. Because of the very gradual onset of the disease, the cognitively healthier spouse hardly realizes that he or she is providing this support and cover. Added to that, of course, is the understandable denial that is likely to have been present, and it is not surprising that no one may have had any awareness of the developing cognitive problems of the survivor.

What are the concerns that family members should have regarding the person with cognitive impairment who lives alone? That varies, of course, depending on whether or not members of the Alzheimer's family are living close by and how often they are able to visit the house to assist and to observe. If no family members are nearby, arrangements will need to be made to have a friend, neighbor, or paid caregiver stop by on a regular basis. However, there are several common areas of concern.

Eating

Is the person with Alzheimer's preparing food and eating it? Only people whose disease is still quite mild are able to shop for groceries, prepare, and consume healthful and well-balanced meals on their own, without assistance. At the least, family members may need to be involved in obtaining groceries, particularly if the individual is no longer driving (see below). If the afflicted person is buying his or her own food, it is a good idea to check what is being purchased. Is it mainly snack foods or sweets, or reasonably nutritious foods? Individuals who are still driving and shopping for groceries independently will often strongly resist assistance in this task, but it may be necessary to insist, for health reasons. For someone with Alzheimer's disease who is preparing meals, foods should be simple, precooked, and requiring only simple microwave reheating. Stove use should be strongly discouraged because of the risks of fire if an inappropriate item is placed on a burner or if an item is forgotten on the stove over a hot burner. Meals on Wheels is a good choice in many communities. These are generally prepared at the local senior center and delivered on a daily basis, in time to be consumed as the noon meal. They are simple, but offer balanced nutrition and are inexpensive. Usually a volunteer will deliver the meal each day, ringing the doorbell and handing it directly to the person who answers. This offers another safeguard: if no one answers the door, someone in the family can be notified.

As an alternative or addition to Meals on Wheels, members of the Alzheimer's family may prepare meals in advance which are then frozen and placed in the afflicted person's freezer. It is a good idea for the family member to check that these are actually being consumed. It is not uncommon that the person with Alzheimer's disease will forget the meal is there or will find the task of reheating it in the microwave overwhelming. It is also a good idea for a family member to regularly check the refrigerator for foods or beverages (such as milk) that may have become spoiled. People with Alzheimer's disease may easily forget something that is in the refrigerator, letting it spoil. But they may also eat spoiled food without realizing it, so someone needs to check and dispose of food that may be unsafe.

People with Alzheimer's disease often report that they have little appetite. This may, in part, have to do with the fact that the senses of taste and smell are frequently quite diminished or absent in persons with Alzheimer's, so food does not have the appeal it once did. Also, because people with Alzheimer's tend to be inactive, they burn fewer calories. Often the best way to determine if the afflicted person who lives alone is eating adequately, aside from noting what food is consumed, is to simply monitor the individual's weight. While it is normal to lose a few pounds over a year, if weight seems to be dropping more rapidly, it may signal that the person is simply too impaired to obtain adequate nutrition on his or her own. If that is the case, it may be necessary to arrange for someone from the family, or even a hired caregiver, to prepare the main meal of the day and remain with the afflicted person during the meal to ensure it is eaten. For most people with Alzheimer's, one good nutritious meal a day is sufficient; the individual can eat whatever he or she wants, or not eat at all during the rest of the day, assuming that does not lead to excessive weight loss.

Falls and Other Emergencies

Many older individuals, including those with Alzheimer's disease, are unsteady on their feet. Falling is an all too common phenomenon among senior citizens. Many older individuals who fall are unable to get themselves up off the floor without considerable assistance from another person. For many older individuals living alone, a lifeline may be a good option. A lifeline is a small electronic device with a large button, usually worn on a chain around the neck or like a wristwatch. When the button is pushed, the lifeline will automatically call the police, the local ambulance, a relative, or whoever the individual designates. Lifelines can be lifesavers, certainly; but they are only valuable if it is very likely that the person will have the presence of mind to push the button when an emergency, such as a fall, occurs. Unfortunately, most persons with even relatively mild Alzheimer's disease cannot reliably use such a device. Even if, in a calm, nonemergency moment, the afflicted person can describe how to use the lifeline, in the crisis of a fall or a sudden sickness, the individual will all too often forget it.

When these issues are raised with the people with Alzheimer's disease who have a tendency to fall, they will likely protest that they do not, in fact, fall very often, and that they can always get up independently if a fall does occur, possibly due to faulty memory, helped along by the strong desire of the afflicted person to continue living alone. A much more complex issue is, how many falls per day, or week, or month, are sufficient to lead the family to act? As noted above, this is one of those areas that demands careful judgment, negotiation, and a keen awareness of the balance that needs to be struck between personal autonomy and independence, on the one hand, and safety on the other.

Falling may be one of the more common emergencies that can

occur for the older person with Alzheimer's living alone, but it is certainly not the only one. Any number of issues can arise that may be health related or not. It is impossible to anticipate every possibility, and the Alzheimer's family will need to have some confidence that the afflicted person living alone has some ability to reach out for assistance if that is necessary. No one should be live alone if they are unable to exit the house on their own, should a fire or other emergency occur in the house. In addition, the afflicted individual should retain the ability to use the telephone and have some idea whom to call depending on the situation. For example, in addition to being able to vacate rapidly, the person living alone should know to call 911 if there were a fire or other household emergency, and should know how to dial the phone to do that. Family members can and should periodically test this, by asking the afflicted person what he or she would do if there were a fire. It may also be helpful for the Alzheimer's family to ask about other scenarios, such as what the person would do if chest pain, vomiting, or the like occurred. Without the ability to reach out effectively in an emergency or an urgent situation—which requires not only the ability to use the phone but the presence of mind to doso at such a moment—it may not be safe for the individual to live alone.

Medications

Many, if not most, older individuals take multiple medications, at various times during the day, and people with Alzheimer's disease are no exception (see appendix for more information on pharmacological treatments). Most Alzheimer's patients are incapable of taking their medications reliably without considerable help from others. At a minimum, that means a pillbox with separate compartments for morning, noon, evening, and bedtime, and for each day of the week. Of course, that is only effective if the individual actually knows what day of the week it is. There are a number of electronic devices on the market that are designed to help people remember to take their medications correctly. They are often not helpful for the person with Alzheimer's disease because of their complexity. Similarly, other techniques, such as leaving reminders, or asking the person to mark off the medications taken on a daily sheet or calendar can sometimes be helpful, but often these techniques fail as well. In fact, nothing can replace having a cognitively intact person supervise medication use on a daily basis—including pouring the pills from the containers at the correct time, handing them to the individual with something to drink, and observing that they are swallowed.

If medications are taken multiple times per day, the clinician may want to suggest that the family ask the physician if all of the medications could be given at the same time of day. However, this may not be possible, because certain medications must be taken multiple times during the day, or can only be given in the morning or at night, for example. However, to whatever degree the individual's medication regimen can be simplified, eliminating all but the most necessary medications and grouping those that remain into as few administrations per day as possible will likely help with compliance. Without a careful plan in place, the risk of missing vital medications is very high, but so is the risk of taking medications more often than prescribed.

Wandering

Wandering refers to the tendency of some individuals with Alzheimer's disease to leave the house and get lost. Usually when people wander in this way, they seem to have a particular goal in mind, although it may be a very confused one. Occasionally, they do seem to be merely idly exploring, with no particular goal in mind—true wandering—but they are unable to find the way home or forget where it is they started from, in the first place.

Wandering is a potentially fatal complication of Alzheimer's disease. Every year, many individuals with Alzheimer's wander, and substantial numbers perish, particularly in the colder months. Even wandering a few dozen yards into the woods, or down a little-used dirt road, can be fatal. Everyone who is able to walk is at risk for wandering, although it is impossible to predict if and when an episode of wandering will occur. Having no history of wandering is certainly no guarantee that it will never happen; every person who wanders for the first time has no history of wandering previously. Overall, it is estimated that more than 60% of people with Alzheimer's disease will wander at some point. Someone who rarely goes out of the house and has no inclination to walk any more than absolutely necessary may be less likely to wander than someone who has always enjoyed being outside and likes to go for walks, but even sedentary individuals have certainly been known to wander and get lost.

Any individual who has a tendency to wander and get lost may not be safe living alone. Anyone who is likely to wander—and statistically that means everyone with Alzheimer's disease—should at least have an identification bracelet from the Alzheimer's Association or similar organization, so that if the person should wander and be found, the ID number and telephone number on the bracelet will provide the vital information that is needed to get the wanderer home safely.

Such bracelets, of course, do require that the person be found, and a more worrisome situation is when someone wanders into a wooded or isolated area where there are no other people around to assist. Simple devices such as a latch hook placed high on the door out of the usual line of sight, and perhaps covered with a cloth, can be helpful to keep someone inside who may otherwise get up in the night and wander out of doors. It is critical that any locking devices be easily released, however, in case of fire.

Increasing numbers of devices are now available, based on GPS technology, that will help locate someone who has wandered away. This is an invaluable technological advance that has the potential to prevent many deaths, although it must be remembered that no technology is foolproof. Nevertheless, such a device may make it possible for someone who lives alone to remain at home longer or substantially delay nursing home placement.

Electronic monitoring devices raise privacy concerns for some; but obtaining and using such a device for the person with dementia can be a life-saving investment.

Autonomy, Safety, and Family Anxiety

How much anxiety should the family have to endure to honor the wishes of the person to remain independent? And how guilty should they feel if the afflicted person does fall and sustain an injury, or worse? These are the kinds of questions that every Alzheimer's family needs to face, and there are no right answers. In such an area, there can be controversy over what is the best option, with strongly held, conflicting opinions among members of the family. The reasons for these different opinions may have more to do with family members' own sense of comfort with risk as well as guilt feelings if they are not very actively involved as caregivers. In fact, it often seems that the family members who have the strongest views on the right thing to do in a given circumstance are the ones who are less involved on a day-to-day basis, for geographical or other reasons. In any case, when there is disagreement about a basic issue such as continued living alone, whether because of falling or other, more general concerns, it would be valuable for family members to meet with the clinician to discuss their different views and the reasons for them. It must be emphasized that there is no correct solution to this problem, and that the decision about whether or not the person with Alzheimer's should continue to live alone needs to be the result of careful discussion among all of the involved family members.

Here the clinician can be very helpful in facilitating such a discussion. If a particular family member insists on clinging to a viewpoint that is significantly different from those of other family members, it may be useful for the clinician to spend some time alone with that person, to try to understand better the reasons for his or her position. When an impasse is reached on this issue, it is likely that there are other areas of disagreement as well. It may be necessary for the clinician to move away from the specific issues at hand and to explore the nature of the relationship between the disagreeing family members in the first place.

As noted in Chapter 1, it is not uncommon, unfortunately, that the needs of a loved one with Alzheimer's will become the battleground for an unresolved conflict between the well parent and an adult child, or between siblings. The clinician can play an important role in moderating such discussions. When two opposing viewpoints cannot easily be resolved, the clinician can point out that the family member who is providing the majority of the daily care (assuming there is an imbalance, as is often the case) should probably have a stronger say in what action is taken. However, if it appears overwhelmingly clear to the clinician the afflicted person is unsafe alone, he or she needs to make this point clearly and insist that action be taken immediately.

Of course, there are elders, including those with Alzheimer's disease, who would welcome not living alone, particularly after the death of a spouse, and for those individuals the difficult issue may not be persuading them to give up the independent living situation but arranging an alternative setting with more care. Other elders, however, with or without Alzheimer's disease, will cling fiercely to their independence and absolutely refuse to consider any living arrangement other than remaining, alone, in their own home. For these people, arranging to have help come into the home may be the only alternative, at least initially. If a family member or a hired caregiver is to visit regularly to provide supervision, it may be that a visit every few days is sufficient. For others, a daily visit may be essential, while still others living alone ideally need someone present much if not all of the time. It takes a very good caregiver (professional or family) to know how to spend the day providing passive caregiving (i.e., observing someone with Alzheimer's who does not need help every moment but needs someone around just in case). The good caregiver will engage the person in appropriate activities and will be an enjoyable companion, rather than just waiting for a need to develop. But he or she will also know how to be unobtrusive so that afflicted persons do not feel that they are simply being watched as if they have done something wrong, as they often feel.

BEING HOME ALONE

When individuals with Alzheimer's disease live with family members, the situation is, of course, somewhat different than when they live alone. Yet the same kinds of concerns apply when the Alzheimer's family needs to decide about the safety of leaving the afflicted person in the house alone for a period of time during the day. As with people who live entirely alone, there are no absolutely right or wrong answers, except in extreme situations. It is a matter of assessing risk and making a decision regarding how much risk is acceptable in order to permit the individual to have some degree of autonomy. Most people with Alzheimer's disease object, at least initially, to the notion that someone must be in the house with them at times when family members are away at work or other activities; they will often insist that they are perfectly fine to stay alone for extended periods of time, even when that does not seem to be objectively true.

Family members will often ask about the number of hours a person can be left alone safely, as if there is some guarantee that nothing adverse will happen if the family is away from the house for, say, 2 hours, but that a longer period of time alone is likely to be hazardous. Of course, these questions are impossible to answer. Any adverse event that could occur when the person is home alone could happen within the first few minutes of the family's absence as easily as it could happen many hours later. Again, it is a matter of assessing and managing risk. Logic would indicate that the longer the person is home alone, the more likely something untoward will occur. Beyond that, there are few objective facts to guide the family in this area.

Issues to be considered when deciding how long to leave someone alone include whether or not there is a reliable neighbor next door who could be called upon in an emergency; whether or not the afflicted person can dial 911 on the telephone; and how likely he is to fall or wander. If the family plans to leave the person alone at lunchtime, food can be prepared and left prominently in the refrigerator on the dining table, ready to eat. While there may be some risk to leaving midday pills out, if these are placed in a small cup on the dining table, many people with Alzheimer's will be able to manage them. Even if pills are missed, it may be possible to give them later.

As a general rule, it would seem that someone with Alzheimer's disease should not be left at home more than 8 hours at a time, unless the person would be capable of living alone in the first place. Usually, the amount of time someone is left home alone is less, but can exceed that if the afflicted person lives with an adult child who needs go to work each day. In those cases, it is usually a good idea to have someone nearby who can check on the person if necessary. The primary caregiver ideally should have a work situation that permits emergency calls, and work should be no more than 15 minutes away by car unless a very reliable person lives closer and can be called upon to go the home if there is a problem.

Families should not leave the person with Alzheimer's home alone for more than a short time if the afflicted individual is unable to use the telephone. Someone home alone for a number of hours should certainly be able to call 911, or call the primary caregiver, depending on the situation. These phone numbers should be programmed into a phone with speed dial capability. Phones are available with very large speed dial buttons that can also hold a photograph of the person to be called. This may be very helpful for someone who generally can manage the phone, but might have difficulty in the face of a minor, or major, emergency.

An excellent alternative for many people with Alzheimer's disease is to attend an adult day program so they are not left home alone for long periods of time. These programs are discussed in Chapter 4.

DRIVING

There is probably no area that causes more tension and disagreements between the Alzheimer's family and the afflicted person than driving. In our society, driving is a potent symbol of independence and freedom. Being in the driver's seat means being in control, literally and figuratively. American society has been built around the automobile for the last several generations, at least. The burgeoning of suburban development beginning after the Second World War, the birth and growth of the shopping center, and the gradual decline of the central city as a place to live and work can all be seen as secondary to the automobile. Getting a driver's license is an important rite of passage in adolescence, and getting one's first car is a happy, proud moment that most everyone can clearly remember decades later. Unfortunately, all of the emphasis on the automobile has caused significant problems as well; traffic jams, pollution, our overreliance on foreign fuel sources, and more than 40,000 motor vehicle fatalities annually, to name a few. It is very difficult, from a practical standpoint, to function in many settings without being able to drive. Except in the center of major cities, one simply needs to drive to get most anywhere. This reality certainly contributes to the intense desire of people with Alzheimer's disease to continue driving, probably long past the point when it is safe. Certainly some afflicted individuals voluntarily give up driving, feeling that they are no longer safe on the road, but they are very much in the minority. Most people with Alzheimer's disease are extremely poor at judging their driving ability, invariably overstating their current abilities. This is only partly due to the strong motivation to continue driving; it also has to do with the disease itself significantly impairing the ability to make accurate assessments of one's ability to perform a complex task such as this one.

There are two different but somewhat related concerns about driving—getting lost and having or causing an accident due to impaired driving abilities. In this way, driving may be unlike some of the other safety issues discussed above; it involves not only the safety of the afflicted individual but may involve the safety of others, as well. It is certainly a tragedy when someone with Alzheimer's disease has an automobile accident and is injured or killed; it becomes a tragedy of unimaginable scope when others are injured or killed as well.

Getting Lost

People with Alzheimer's disease often have impaired visuospatial abilities, which involve being able to understand visual representations and spatial relationships between objects. It is likely that the parietal lobes play an important role in spatial analysis and understanding spatial relationships. People with visuospatial problems may have difficulty finding their way from one place to another. In extreme cases, this can happen even within the house, so that afflicted people may literally not be able to find the bathroom, or find their way back to the bedroom after using the toilet during the night. More commonly, and much earlier in the illness, visuospatial problems can lead to getting lost while driving. Routes that should be familiar become foreign to the afflicted person. Being able to follow driving directions from the computer or a map, or even from road signs, becomes difficult or impossible.

It is not uncommon for people with Alzheimer's disease who get lost to drive miles out of their way hoping to find where they are going. Adding to the visuospatial difficulties are poor problem-solving skills, such that even if individuals become aware that they are lost, they may not know how to deal with the problem in a sensible way (like stopping to ask directions). They may even forget where they were going in the first place. In addition, when people with Alzheimer's disease do realize that they have gotten lost while driving, they are likely to panic, and to drive more erratically as a result. This connects the first problem in driving with Alzheimer's disease—getting lost—with the second problem: dangerous driving. When drivers are frightened, panicked, angry, or merely very confused, the safety of their driving decreases markedly. Lanes are changed without signaling; left-hand turns are made from the right lane; speed may be excessively slow or fast, and there is generally less attentiveness to the road and to other vehicles.

Even when people with Alzheimer's disease do not get lost, the quality of their driving may be significantly impaired. It has been shown that they are less attentive to street signs, will get too close to one side of a lane or the other, and will drift into the next lane unexpectedly. Visuospatial difficulties can cause an inability to judge how far the curb is from the wheels of the car, or how far other vehicles are on either side or in front or behind. Turn signals are forgotten, and braking can be excessively sudden, or delayed, causing rear or front end collisions, respectively. Afflicted individuals may drive the wrong way on a one-way street, or around a rotary, or press the gas pedal when they intended to press the brake. People with Alzheimer's are much less able to react quickly if a nearby car is driving unsafely, or if a dog or a small child should dart into the street.

These difficulties generally begin quite gradually, so that the person with the disease, and even the spouse, may not be aware of them until a problem develops. A minor accident, such as brushing a parked car or a road sign, can be dismissed or rationalized all too easily. The problem can be compounded when the person with Alzheimer's disease is married to someone who has never driven and who therefore relies on her spouse (usually the nondriver is a woman) for transportation. Both members of the couple now have a strong motivation not to find any fault with the person's driving.

Unfortunately, the problem with driving is commonly recognized only after a serious event has occurred; either a frightening episode of getting lost, which may have required police intervention, or an accident. Even after such an event, the individual may be very reluctant to stop driving. This position is aided by significant denial, poor judgment, and simply not recalling the accident a few days later.

Occasionally, it is clear that someone who is driving should no longer be doing so. There have been accidents, episodes of getting lost, and the person no longer understands the meaning of a stop sign. In such cases, if the family has not yet acted definitively to put an end to the person's driving, they must do so immediately, and if there is stalling on this, the clinician will need to take a firm stand and make suggestions for how to approach the problem. Family members may feel intimidated by the afflicted person, and are irrationally fearful of doing anything that will cause offense or anger. This often reflects the nature of the relationship prior to Alzheimer's. The individual who is now afflicted with disease may always have been in charge in the family and may have ruled with subtle or not-so-subtle intimidation, while spouse and children were submissive. Yet it is absolutely necessary to prevent someone who is hazardous on the road from continuing to drive. In addition to confronting the individual with the realities of the situation, it may be necessary to take the car keys, disable the car, or—better—remove it. Faced with this, people with Alzheimer's may even go so far as to attempt to purchase another car: that is how vitally important driving is and how poorly people are able to judge their own abilities or respond to the advice that is given. When this happens, it is certainly advisable to have a visit with the physician, who should tell the person that he or she cannot drive.

In most states, it is not illegal to drive with Alzheimer's disease, but it may be useful for the physician to point out that a recommendation not to drive has been recorded in the medical record. Now, should there be an accident, insurance may refuse to cover the person because he or she was driving against medical advice Whether or not this would actually occur, it may nevertheless be a useful stance the physician may use to achieve an end that is certainly justified. It is also incumbent upon the physician to notify the state motor vehicle bureau immediately of the recommendations and urge that the person's license be suspended until repeat testing can be done. Some states require a written test before the road test can be given, and many persons with Alzheimer's disease will fail the written test even if they might have passed the road test. This is simply because passing a written test relies on recent memory, whereas driving also involves some elements of procedural memory that may remain sufficiently intact to help the person with Alzheimer's pass a simple road test. Most state road examinations are not difficult, and do not involve unexpected situations where the driver needs to act quickly to avoid an accident. Thus patients who only have to pass a road test occasionally can do so when common sense indicates that they should definitely not be driving. While the fact of passing the motor vehicle test may lessen the burden of responsibility on the family or even the physician, the problem is now magnified because the individual can now point out that the state felt it was permissible for him to drive. Thus the family who feels intimidated by the afflicted person's insistence on driving cannot necessarily rely on the motor vehicle bureau to solve the problem. It can sometimes be helpful to alert local police to the situation, in detail, and ask that they be especially watchful for and ticket any infractions, but even this is not always successful because local police cannot be expected to watch the afflicted person's driving at all times.

The Driving Intervention

Of course, the best solution is for the family to persuade the individual to give up driving voluntarily, hopefully before there are serious consequences. It may be necessary to convene the family for an intervention similar to that discussed in Chapter 3, as an attempt to deal with denial of illness. Certainly the belief that one can drive when it is no longer safe to do so is the result of a severe degree of denial, in addition to simple unawareness regarding one's difficulties. It is critical that all participants in the intervention be in agreement about the situation. If nearly everyone in the family feels the person should not drive, but one family member feels that very limited driving with another person in the car is acceptable, that more permissive view is all the afflicted individual will be likely to hear or remember. More than one intervention may be necessary. The clinician can be very helpful in suggesting the need for this intervention and in guiding family members as to the most effective approaches to take. It is often useful for the clinician to clarify the feelings that are behind the family member's reluctance to confront the person with Alzheimer's disease.

At times, incremental changes in driving, rather than a total cessation, may be reasonable. Perhaps it is felt that the individual cannot drive alone but that going with a family member in the passenger seat is acceptable. This would most often apply when the problem has more to do with getting lost than the quality of driving. Another incremental step may be that the person should not drive at night, or when there is snow on the road, or on a four-lane highway, or anywhere except a few blocks to town and back. While there really is no evidence that such restrictions reduce the risk of accidents, common sense would suggest that they may be appropriate under limited circumstances. However, knowing that Alzheimer's disease is progressive and that driving skills can certainly change over a short period of time, if such an incremental step is taken, it will be necessary to revisit the decision frequently. Regular reevaluation of driving safety needs to be part of any agreement with the family if any driving is to continue.

How does the family keep watch on the driving of the person who has Alzheimer's disease? Certainly they cannot rely on self-reports. Nor should they assume that if there have been no accidents, no tickets, or no major episodes of getting lost, everything is fine. The only way to judge driving ability is to drive with someone, either in the same car or in another car following close behind. People with Alzheimer's disease usually resent having their driving observed in this way, but it is essential. Ideally, different family members should ride with or closely follow the person with Alzheimer's disease, to get the most comprehensive picture of driving ability.

Except in the extreme cases, the memory specialist is not in a position to determine whether or not driving is safe. Unfortunately, there are no office tests that inform this issue. While tests of visuospatial abilities, such as clock drawing, may be correlated with how likely it is that the person with Alzheimer's disease will get lost while driving, the correlation is not high, and performance on such a test is not predictive of overall driving safety. One of the best ways to determine whether or not it is safe for someone who has Alzheimer's disease to continue to drive is the "grandchild test." If the person in question has young grandchildren, the grandchild's parents—the afflicted person's son, daughter, son-in-law, or daughter-in-law—should be asked if they would allow their young child to ride with the grandparent. If the answer is no, the person simply should not drive.

It is not enough for the family to get someone with Alzheimer's disease to agree to stop driving, as important as that is. The family must also make it very clear how they will take over those tasks that previously were done by the afflicted person using a car. Family members need to arrange to drive the person where he or she needs and wants to go, or make arrangements for others to provide the transportation. It is usually not a very satisfying compromise to the individual with Alzheimer's disease to be told, "We'll take you wherever you want to go," but it may help to some degree, and it is certainly necessary to plan how trips will take place.

CHAPTER 7

Dealing With Mood
and Behavioral Issues

❖ In Alzheimer's disease, it is estimated that more than 90% of afflicted people (Marin et al., 1997) will have one or more significant mood or behavioral symptoms at some point during the course of their illness. Any behavioral problem can occur at nearly any point in the disease, but behavioral symptoms that occur typically in early Alzheimer's include apathy, depression, anxiety, insomnia, and irritability; later in the disease, additional symptoms include agitation, paranoia, disinhibition, agitation, and aggressiveness toward others. It should be remembered that Alzheimer's is a neuropsychiatric disease, not simply a medical or neurological condition.

Mood and behavioral symptoms certainly increase the suffering of both the afflicted individual and the Alzheimer's family. These symptoms decrease functional abilities and occasionally lead to dangerous behaviors. An example might be a husband with Alzheimer's who becomes so convinced that his elderly wife is having an affair that he becomes physically aggressive toward her. Numerous studies have shown that poorly controlled behavioral symptoms are a major cause of hastened nursing home placement. It is these behavioral symptoms, more than almost anything, that drain the resources of caregivers, however loving and devoted they may be.

Why do behavioral problems occur with such frequency? They develop because of the brain damage that is caused by the disease process itself; in that sense they are no different than the memory loss, language disturbance, loss of ability to perform daily tasks, and other symptoms that are at the heart of the disease. In addition, however, certain behavioral syndromes can develop as a psychological reaction to the disease (frustration, sadness, or anger, for example), particularly in the earlier stages.

Some of the basic characteristics of Alzheimer's disease that can lead to mood and behavioral symptoms are the following:

- **Loss of inhibition and impulse control.** This characteristic is due to damage in the frontal parts of the brain and its connections, and is extremely common in Alzheimer's disease and some of the other dementias. People with loss of inhibition act on impulse; they may say or do things without being concerned about the impact on others; and they express, through words and behaviors, their emotional reactions to situations rather than being able to control them in more socially appropriate ways. People with damage in the frontal lobes of the brain may be unaware of, or unconcerned about, the concepts of right and wrong.

- **Loss of mood regulation.** This is due to damage in vital areas of the brain and can lead to depression, manic behaviors, frequent changes in emotions (emotional lability), or the tendency to display every emotion openly.

- **Decreased comprehension of the immediate environment, which can lead to misperceptions, misunderstanding, and strong reactions.** For example, people with Alzheimer's may misperceive the intent of a home health aide and feel that this individual who is trying to assist them with bathing is actually trying to assault them physically or sexually.

- **Frustration.** It goes without saying that it is extraordinarily frustrating for the person with Alzheimer's disease to suffer from such a poor memory and impaired ability to carry out tasks, no matter how much or little conscious awareness there is regarding these limitations. Extreme frustration, particularly in someone who has also lost impulse control, can lead to a variety of difficult behaviors.

- **Poor judgment**. Because of damage to frontal lobe systems, persons with Alzheimer's disease frequently lose the ability to make sound judgments about even trivial matters as well as more significant ones. The effect of this, like the effect of loss of inhibition and impulse control, can be to turn a formerly calm, pleasant, and thoughtful person into someone who can be very challenging interpersonally.

- **Catastrophic reactions**. Mace and Rabins (2006), in *The 36-Hour Day*, use this term (borrowed from earlier literature on traumatic brain injury) to describe an emotional overreaction in someone with Alzheimer's disease when confronted with a stimulus that is too complex, noxious, new, or confusing, or a task that is too difficult for the individual. When faced with this situation, the person with Alzheimer's disease becomes excessively angry, upset, anxious, frightened, irritable, or aggressive, as an involuntary response to the unpleasant stimulus. As persons become more demented, they are increasingly prone to these emotional overreactions, stimulated by what may at time seem like trivial events. The concept of a catastrophic reaction is very useful in learning how to understand the sometimes puzzling behaviors of persons with Alzheimer's disease and other dementias. It can also help the caregiver think of ways to avoid similar reactions in the future, by analyzing and understanding the apparent precipitant and avoiding it if possible.

- **"He's doing it on purpose!"** At times, certain behaviors of the person with Alzheimer's disease seem purposeful, or intentional, as if they are being done simply to annoy the caregiver. Putting things in odd places or being unable to get dressed independently are examples. The behavior may appear volitional because there is such variability from day to day or even from hour to hour. Simply because someone was able to do something on her own yesterday does not mean that she can do the same thing today. In addition, individuals with Alzheimer's disease frequently become unable to appreciate other people's feelings or needs as sensitively as they once did. As a result, they can seem selfish or self-centered and uncaring about other people. In reality, they are unable to recognize others' needs or feelings, because of the disease. In general, when trying to determine whether someone with Alzheimer's disease cannot do a particular task or simply will not do the task (implying some degree of choice), one should always assume that he or she cannot do the task now, even if he or she could do it yesterday, or last week, or even earlier today. Even if that assumption is not always correct, it is a stance that leads to less friction and anger on the part of the caregiver. After all, the goal is not necessarily to uncover the ultimate truth about a complex behavior or interaction but to simply get through the day with as little stress as possible, both for the person with Alzheimer's and for the members of the Alzheimer's family.

THE EFFECT OF THE UNDERLYING PERSONALITY

One's personality type before developing Alzheimer's disease may play a role in determining the mood and behavioral symptoms that appear after Alzheimer's or a related disorder develops. For example, someone who has always been high-strung and a worrier is likely to suffer significant anxiety with the disease. A person who was always somewhat suspicious of others may well become paranoid once Alzheimer's disease sets in. Persons who are "control freaks"—Type As who need to be in charge—often have a very difficult time with the disease, because Alzheimer's and the impairments it produces take away the ability to be in control in many fundamental ways; but the disease does not necessarily lessen the individual's desire or need to be in control. On the other hand, persons who are easygoing, somewhat passive, and glad to have others be in control and make decisions for them often have an easier time dealing with Alzheimer's disease.

There are certainly exceptions to this. Someone who was very difficult before Alzheimer's disease may become much easier to get along with; conversely, people sometimes develop difficult characteristics that are quite different than their earlier very pleasant character style. There is no way of predicting or controlling the kinds of personality traits that may develop as part of Alzheimer's disease. It may have more to do with the specific areas of the brain that are most severely affected by the disease (which is different from person to person) than anything else.

Relationship Issues

People who have unresolved conflicts in their marriage (or parent-child relationship if a child is the primary caregiver) may have more difficulty in the caregiving situation than those who began the illness journey with a better relationship. Inevitably, some of the unresolved issues that may have been avoided for years, or decades, will come to the surface. However, behavioral and interpersonal issues can develop even in the context of the strongest relationships; the quality of the relationship will only make the situation better, or worse, but will not totally eliminate some of the behavioral challenges that develop when someone has Alzheimer's disease.

At times, the onset of Alzheimer's disease and a new caregiving role can lead to fundamental growth and improvement in a marital or parent-child relationship that was previously mired in dysfunction. The clinician can play an important role in helping to bring about these changes.

COPING WITH BEHAVIORS

The clinician should encourage family members to examine the behavior. There should always be an assumption that there is a reason why a difficult behavior occurred exactly when and how it did. Trying to make sense out of something that may seem senseless is not always successful, but it can often lead to a better understanding of the needs of the person with Alzheimer's disease and may help avoid the problem the next time. It can also help the caregiver feel less passive and victimized by the behaviors to adopt an attitude of curiosity about their meaning. Clinicians should ask family members to consider the following "W questions" in response to an episode of difficult behavior:

- With *whom* did the behavior occur?
- *When* did it occur?
- *Where* did it occur?
- *What* was the context of the behavior?
- *Why* did it occur?

For example, Mr. Jones's agitation had become a problem. He yelled, cursed, and on one occasion pinched his caregiver, Beth. His wife called the physician asking for medication to deal with it. However, in discussing the incident using the W questions, some possible solutions other than medication became apparent:

- *With whom?* Mr. Jones became agitated only with one particular caregiver, Beth. This did not happen when the alternate caregiver, Susan, was with him.
- *When?* He was generally calm all day until about 8 P.M., when these behaviors tended to occur.
- *Where?* The most intense agitation occurred in the bathroom.
- *What was the context?* Beth was trying to assist him with showering, before bedtime.

It may be difficult to determine with certainty exactly why a behavior occurred, but often the reason can be deduced from the answers to the W questions. In this case, it seems clear that Mr. Jones's agitation has to do with being showered by Beth. Several possible solutions should be considered before resorting to medication. Perhaps Beth's approach to Mr. Jones needs to be examined. Does she rush him? Does her attempt to get him showered seem overly forceful? Even if they are not intended that way, certainly, could her behaviors be interpreted by him as aggressive? Also, he is showering at a time when many people with Alzheimer's disease have little frustration tolerance—bedtime. Perhaps a shower earlier in the day would work better. If not, perhaps Susan, the alternate caregiver, has a gentler approach since there is no report of his becoming aggressive with her. Alternatively, perhaps a bath or even a sponge bath would be less upsetting to him. Thus, reviewing the W questions surrounding an episode of agitation helps uncover a cause for the behavioral outbursts and may suggest several possible solutions.

In reviewing a catastrophic reaction or other difficult behavioral event, it is important to consider what is in the environment, the routine, or the family's behavior that needs to change to reduce the likelihood of a similar event in the future. The clinician should emphasize that the environment, the routine, or the family is not to blame for what has happened, but that the person with Alzheimer's disease cannot be expected to learn new ways of reacting, so the others need to be the ones to change. People with Alzheimer's disease are largely incapable of new learning or modifying their behavior simply because they have been asked to do so, no matter how agreeable they were previously. In the example given above, each of the solutions proposed for dealing with Mr. Jones's agitation involves changing something in the environment, and not trying to change Mr. Jones by telling him to behave or giving him medication. Of course, under certain circumstances, medications may be a very useful adjunct in treating behavioral disturbances, but they should not be used in place of modifications to the environment or improvements in how the caregiver interacts with the person with Alzheimer's.

The Importance of Routine

Novel situations make persons with Alzheimer's disease uncomfortable, and even something new that seems like a positive change of pace can trigger a catastrophic reaction. Sameness and predictability day in and day out are very comforting for people with memory disorders, even if that sameness would have been excruciating prior to the illness. This is especially important to remember around the holidays, when new situations with lots of stimulation were once exciting and enjoyable but now can lead to a very unpleasant time for all concerned.

Distraction

One of the most useful tools in dealing with difficult situations is to distract the person or change the topic of conversation. For example, when the individual brings up questions such as "When will I drive again?" or "Where is my mother?," giving a vague response and then quickly changing the topic to one less emotionally charged is a valuable tool. The clinician may want to review different scenarios with the family member, helping to identify topics that are likely to be highly charged for the person with Alzheimer's disease, and suggesting topics that can be brought up as a distraction. One small consolation of short-term memory loss is that successful distraction may cause the person to forget whatever he or she was concerned about moments earlier, because of the introduction of a new topic. At times these issues are of such importance that the person cannot be distracted, but this technique works surprisingly frequently. Being good at distraction takes creativity and being able to think on your feet and may not come naturally at first, but is a technique that can be learned with practice. The clinician should role-play the part of the person with Alzheimer's disease and help the family member practice responding quickly with less charged subjects.

Activities

Often, it is best to distract someone with an activity, rather than just conversation, particularly as the disease progresses and meaningful conversation becomes more difficult. The clinician may suggest examples of activities that are frequently helpful in calming a person with Alzheimer's disease:

- Listening to music
- Going for a walk to look at nature
- Taking a ride in the car
- Watching animal, travel, nature, or cooking shows on television
- Having a massage
- Preparing and eating comfort food together
- Other activities that are primarily focused on the senses and are not verbally based.

These activities can remain effective and pleasurable long after verbal communication becomes a significant challenge. Listening to music can be particularly valuable, if someone previously enjoyed music and likes the type of music played.

MANAGING AGGRESSION

Some verbal aggressiveness (even from someone formerly very mild mannered) should be seen as an almost inevitable part of the illness. The clinician should help the family member not to take it personally and not to react in kind. More serious verbal aggression and physical aggression are less frequent in persons with Alzheimer's disease but do occur, and need to be taken very seriously. Aggressive outbursts can be viewed as the result of a number of different factors in someone with Alzheimer's disease:

- Loss of judgment and the sense of social appropriateness
- Loss of impulse control
- Frustration over one's own limitations
- Frustration over the limitations of autonomy placed on the individual as a result of the illness
- Depression or irritability
- Misperceiving someone who is trying to help as someone who is trying to harm
- Catastrophic reactions
- Misdirected responses to physical pain or distress
- Many others

Abusiveness, severe verbal aggressiveness, or any degree of physical aggression toward a person or property calls for immediate action. The clinician must emphasize that caregivers must protect their own safety, first and foremost. Depending on the situation, an aggressive episode may require an urgent consultation with the physician or a call to 911. Many emergency responders are aware and sensitive to the fact that aggressive outbursts can occur in persons with Alzheimer's disease and will try to help settle the situation, ensure the safety of the victim, and possibly arrange to have the person evaluated by the local emergency room.

For the Alzheimer's family member, it is certainly appropriate to very clearly indicate to the individual that such behavior is completely unacceptable, but doing so may not have a lasting effect, due to the memory disorder. The clinician may need to encourage a previously submissive spouse or adult child to be quite firm about this; clearly, controlling aggression is in everyone's best interest, including that of the person with Alzheimer's disease. Repeated episodes of aggressiveness are one of the most frequent precipitants for placement in a long-term care facility.

Certainly, any episode of physical aggression should be a clear call for some significant change in the caregiving situation, including the following:

- Clear messages to the person that such behaviors cannot be tolerated
- Consideration of more outside assistance
- An urgent consultation with the physician, to review whether or not medication treatment for aggressiveness might be appropriate
- A review of what may have led to the aggressive episode, to determine what environmental changes might be helpful to prevent such behaviors in the future

Once again, the clinician may want to emphasize that reviewing the episode to see what might be done differently in the future does not imply that the caregiver must have been at fault for what occurred, but that it is only the caregiver, and not the person with Alzheimer's disease, who may be able to make some behavioral change that will lessen the likelihood of similar episodes occurring in the future. Of course, it is possible that something in the caregiver's behavior did contribute to the episode. It can be very challenging for the clinician to explore this area without seeming to blame the caregiver for what happened, and a great deal of tact is needed, particularly with family members who already feel guilty about their interactions with the afflicted person, or caregivers who are angry and defensive and feel excessively put upon by the behaviors of the person with the disease. Nevertheless, valuable learning can come from recognizing, in retrospect, what one did that might have prompted aggressive behavior in the person with Alzheimer's disease.

Medications that can be considered for aggressiveness are discussed in the appendix.

MANAGING ANXIETY

If the person with Alzheimer's disease was previously an anxious or dependent person, then it is likely that he or she will continue to be anxious or dependent, perhaps even more so. Most often, anxiety in the person with Alzheimer's disease has to do with being afraid of not being able to care for oneself, although commonly the individual is not consciously aware of that or able to express those feelings directly. Instead, their behaviors may involve shadowing, which entails following the caregiver everywhere, so the caregiver is never out of sight. This can be quite challenging for the caregiver, particularly when the need for closeness continues into the bathroom and other inappropriate settings.

Some anxiety is common in people with Alzheimer's disease, as the individual gains some awareness of the cognitive losses. Later in the illness, as this awareness fades, anxiety can in fact lessen.

For persons who were never anxious or dependent prior to having Alzheimer's disease, significant anxiety could actually signal an underlying depression. It would be a good idea for the afflicted person's physician to be consulted if there is concern about such a change in demeanor.

Other people with Alzheimer's disease who develop significant anxiety may actually need more day-to-day structure or support; their anxiety may be a signal that they can no longer manage the degree of independence they have (even though they may still express a strong desire for that independence).

For most persons with Alzheimer's disease, and certainly those who have a great deal of anxiety, telling the individual about plans or events coming up in the future may only cause an increase in fretting and innumerable repetitive questions about the event. In these circumstances, it may be best to not announce upcoming plans until there is a need to know (i.e., right before the event).

This may not seem kind, or fair, since that is not how these issues would have been handled in the past, but it is important to remember that the kindest, fairest way to treat someone with Alzheimer's disease is usually to do what will cause them the least distress.

Medications for treating anxiety are discussed in the appendix.

MANAGING APATHY

As noted in Chapter 5, apathy is defined as diminished motivation. Persons who have apathy have a decreased or absent ability or desire to initiate any activity. Apathy is one of the most common but also one of the most misunderstood symptoms in Alzheimer's disease. It is often seen as something else—overmedication, medical illness, depression, or even laziness.

While it is possible, of course, that the person with Alzheimer's has been overmedicated or is suffering from a physical ailment that causes excessive fatigue, it may simply be that the individual naps frequently because of apathy. When there is no motivation or internal drive to be engaged in activity, it is very easy for the older individual to spend much of the day napping off and on. If, during a day that is particularly active, the person with Alzheimer's disease is able to remain alert all day, overmedication is probably not the issue. People with apathy rise to the occasion and usually do not seem sleepy when they are stimulated or engaged.

Differentiating Apathy From Depression

Apathy can easily be mistaken for depression. But there are some questions that will help the clinician differentiate the two. Persons who are apathetic but not depressed will be able to enjoy an activity if it is presented to them, but left to their own devices they might not be likely to pursue it. For example, apathetic individuals might seem very content sitting on the couch all day, and might say no when asked if they want to go out for lunch. But if they are persuaded to go, they may thoroughly enjoy the experience and will often express pleasure at having participated. However, the person with apathy will not learn from that experience that it is more enjoyable to do things than to sit passively.

Someone who is depressed but not apathetic does not appear to want to pursue activities, either. The depressed individual, when taken to lunch or another activity, does not really enjoy the activity but may simply "go through the motions." Usually the lack of pleasure is readily apparent. While this explanation may make it seem as if it is simple to differentiate these two states, in practice it can sometimes be difficult to tell the difference between apathy and depression.

The clinician can play an important role in helping the caregiver understand apathy properly and not be disturbed by it or angry for this change in behavior over which the individual has absolutely no control. It is not laziness, but a result of brain disease. As noted in Chapter 5, structuring activities for the person with Alzheimer's disease is critical, since the afflicted individual is unable to do this independently. Medication for apathy is discussed in the appendix.

REPETITIVE QUESTIONS

Asking the same question over and is one of the hallmark symptoms of early Alzheimer's disease. While not in the same category as other behavioral symptoms discussed here, the caregiver's reaction can be similar to other difficult behaviors. Only the most patient of caregivers is able to maintain equanimity in the face of being asked the same question again and again in a short period of time.

Often caregivers are doubly stressed, first by the impact of the repetitive questioning, and second, by the enormous guilt they feel after getting angry at their loved one for asking the same question over and over. Here, it can be helpful for the clinician to remind caregivers that repetitive questioning is a core symptom of the disease, since it is a direct effect of short-term memory impairment, and therefore there is absolutely no way to avoid it. In addition, it is helpful to point out that persons with Alzheimer's disease have an even greater tendency to ask repetitive questions when the topic is something that makes them anxious. Thus, if the person with Alzheimer's asks even more incessantly than usual about when company is coming for dinner, there is a good possibility that he or she is anxious about the visit. While there is little likelihood that the person would be able to acknowledge that anxiety, a reassuring comment that it will only be a short visit with old, dear friends might help to decrease the anxiety and therefore the questions.

Finally, it is valuable to reassure the guilty caregiver that it is nearly impossible to be in the caregiving role for any length of time without having an occasional loss of temper. If these episodes occur with increasing frequency or intensity, however, it may mean that the caregiver needs more help and more time free of caregiving entirely (respite). At worst, it could be a sign of developing caregiver burnout or abuse, and more drastic action may be necessary (see Chapter 8). It is important for the clinician to inquire specifically about these episodes, since members of the Alzheimer's family are often embarrassed to bring up episodes of becoming angry or losing their temper. In general, it is important for the clinician to try to establish a relationship of trust in which the caregiver will feel comfortable expressing feelings and reactions without worrying about being judged. Being able to talk about the strong feelings that have been generated by aspects of the caregiving experience, without fear of being judged, will help lower the caregiver's stress considerably.

MANAGING DELUSIONS AND OTHER FALSE BELIEFS

Delusions are fixed, false beliefs. By definition, someone cannot be talked out of a delusion or have it broken down by logical arguments. Delusions occur in a large percentage of persons with Alzheimer's disease. They can also occur in other purely psychiatric conditions, such as schizophrenia or bipolar illness.

In someone with Alzheimer's disease, it may be unclear if a false belief is due to a psychotic process or to the cognitive disorder itself. Significant Alzheimer's disease can cause the individual to be unable to stay focused on objective current reality. He or she may confuse the past with the present, or confuse a thought or a wish or dream with a real event. Such beliefs may not be true delusions. However, more important than how we label these symptoms is to determine whether or not the beliefs are disturbing to the individual, or others, or interfering in some way with functioning. They require urgent attention if they lead to dangerous behaviors or cause significant distress (e.g., feeling that one's young child is lost when, in fact, all the children are grown and long out of the house). If, however, beliefs are benign and not upsetting to the person, then no intervention is needed, and there is no reason to correct the mistaken belief.

Some common false beliefs in Alzheimer's disease follow:

- **"My parents are still alive."** If people are not distressed by thinking their parents are alive but do not visit, then there is no point in trying to reorient them to current reality. It can be repeatedly upsetting every time people are told that their parents are deceased (even when this happened decades earlier). It is likely that such a belief reflects the need and desire to have the comfort of one's parents, because cognitive impairment leaves these individuals feeling vulnerable, unprotected, perhaps lonely, and somewhat like a child. Caregivers should try not to convince their loved one about the reality of the parent's death. Going over how old the parents would be if they were still alive, or showing the person death certificates is only upsetting or confusing, and at best will be effective for the moment only; later in the same day, or the next day, the delusion may return. It is best to deal with it by distraction and reassurance that even if the parents aren't there right now, the caregiver is there to provide whatever help the person needs. It is only a good idea to gently remind people that their parents are no longer living if they are very distressed with worrying about them, wondering if anything bad has happened to them, or feeling abandoned because the parents no longer visit. This common belief is generally not responsive to medication treatment, although if an afflicted person is continuously and significantly upset by the belief that his parents have abandoned him, or some similar negative thought, careful assessment for depression should be performed, and if necessary depression should be treated (see next section).
- **"I do all the housework at home."** This belief may be a mis-

taken memory (or a memory from years ago, not from the present). It may also represent the desire of the person to appear more functional. It is often associated with a significant amount of denial. There is no reason to challenge this belief, even though caregivers may understandably feel annoyed that they actually do all the work at home, but the person with Alzheimer's disease is taking all the credit. Setting the reality straight just leads to defensiveness and arguments, and there is no reason to do that.

- **"My husband/wife has another woman/man."** This is a surprisingly common belief in both men and women with Alzheimer's disease. It may reflect a fear that the person is no longer desirable or lovable, and that the spouse would be better off with someone else who is not such a burden. This belief can also reflect unresolved dynamics in a marital relationship or may even grow from actual events in the past. It is important to state the reality, although it will likely need to be repeated frequently.

- **"Someone is stealing my things."** This symptom usually reflects a significant degree of denial, and is people's somewhat paranoid response to the fact that (as is common in Alzheimer's disease) they have misplaced personal belongings somewhere in the house or cannot remember what they did or did not own. Persons who develop this delusional belief may have a need to blame others rather than seeing the problem as related to their own forgetfulness. Dealing with the symptom depends on how distressing or pervasive the belief is. Certainly, it does no good to insist that the items were not stolen. Instead, it is always more helpful for the caregiver to simply assist the person in trying to find what is missing. Often, it involves items that are valued by the person, which have been hidden away in a quickly forgotten location. Sometimes, the items would have no value to others, such as a toothbrush or an old slipper. Those items may eventually be found in unexpected locations (e.g., the toothbrush may be in the freezer or the pocket of a raincoat hanging in the hall closet). Medications are not likely to be helpful with this problem.

- **"Someone is trying to harm me."** This delusion is usually very distressing for the individual and can lead to very difficult situations with the Alzheimer's family. Often the individual with Alzheimer's believes that it is the primary caregiver or another family member who wants to cause harm. It may or may not reflect underlying tensions in the caregiver relationship; the belief can develop in relationships that have previously been very strong. If the symptoms are severe and causing a great deal of distress, medication may be considered (see Chapter 3).

- **"You aren't my wife/husband."** This is a common belief that develops in persons with Alzheimer's disease. Understandably, it is very upsetting to both members of the couple. While it may have delusional components, it actually reflects an agnosia, which is a general term for a loss of ability to recognize objects or people who should be familiar. It is not that the spouse is forgotten; the person with Alzheimer's can no longer connect the visual, auditory, or other signals from the spouse with those parts of the brain that remember the spouse, so the person looks like a stranger. Women who have this agnosia may say, "Have you seen my husband?" or something similar, making it clear that the spouse is still remembered and missed.

    Dealing with the inability of someone to recognize the spouse can be challenging. As usual, it does no good to confront the afflicted individual with reality, or to try to prove who the spouse is by showing a marriage certificate or some such. However, it is understandable that spouses will want to make their identity very clear, whether or not it helps. Using distraction, changing the subject, or comments such as, "I'm sure he'll be back soon" may help, although often the person will be persistent. It may help for the caregiver to leave the room and come back a few minutes later; surprisingly, upon his or her return, the individual may have no problem recognizing the person accurately, and usually will not recall the "other" person who had seemingly been present moments earlier. Another technique that sometimes helps is to wear an old piece of clothing that has meaning in the relationship (perhaps a distinctive shirt given to the spouse by the person many years ago) or a cologne (if he or she retains the ability to perceive odors) that was worn throughout the marriage. This is generally not a symptom that suddenly appears and remains fixed; during what can be a long phase of losing the ability to recognize the spouse, the individual may go from moment to moment recognizing and not recognizing the spouse. This is confusing, exasperating, and upsetting for the spouse. The main task in dealing with this is not to be upset by the agnosia. The best outcome of this situation may be that the person with Alzheimer's comes to realize that this person who is always around is a very good new friend, even while having no idea of his or her actual identity. Agnosias of this kind are generally not responsive to medication.

- **"This place is not my house."** The person with Alzheimer's disease is unable to make a connection between the visual and other stimuli created by being in the house and the actual brain memory of their home. In addition, afflicted individuals may remember a home they lived in many years before, and do not remember the current house, particularly if they have lived there for only a relatively short time. Less commonly, people with Alzheimer's disease will lose the ability to recognize their own image in a mirror and will be frightened, angered, or upset by the presence of an intruder in their home. This agnosia can be so upsetting that it becomes necessary to remove the mirrors from the house.

Agnosias are not helped by any psychotropic medications, although if someone becomes extremely agitated by, for example, believing intruders are in the home, an as-needed dose of medication for agitation could be helpful. Medications for agitation are discussed in the appendix.

MANAGING DEPRESSION

Depression is one of the most common mood and behavioral complications of Alzheimer's disease. It can be understood it two ways: as a brain illness, due to damage in those areas of the brain that control mood, and also as a psychological reaction to the enormous losses that result from the disease. Both views are accurate and are complementary.

Although a large percentage of people with Alzheimer's disease develop significant depressive symptoms, it can be difficult to make a diagnosis of depression, for a number of reasons. Older individuals often have a variety of physical symptoms that may be similar to certain symptoms of depression (e.g., fatigue, loss of energy, poor concentration, preoccupation with aches and pains) and so the symptoms of depression may be mistakenly attributed to the individual's chronic physical illnesses. People with Alzheimer's disease who have depression are often not able to clearly express their internal mood state, if indeed they even are aware of it; many older persons, demented or not, who have depression will deny feeling sadness, for a variety of reasons. People with Alzheimer's disease will frequently express depression in somewhat indirect ways; rather than talking about feeling unhappy, they will be irritable or even aggressive toward others.

One of the most reliable indicators of depression in the person with Alzheimer's disease is the presence of *anhedonia*, or the inability to experience pleasure. This may not be total, depending on the severity of depression; there may be a diminished sense of enjoyment with activities that once were pleasurable. Individuals appear to merely be "going through the motions;" they may derive some pleasure from a particular activity, but much less than at an earlier time when they were not depressed. As noted before, it is important to distinguish apathy from depression, although this can be challenging at times, and both can be present at the same time.

One concern in anyone with significant depression is suicide. Fortunately, it is quite rare for people with Alzheimer's disease to attempt suicide, even if they said at an earlier stage in life, "If I ever get Alzheimer's disease, I'll kill myself." What is common, however, is for people with Alzheimer's disease to state that they wish they would die, or that they should die, because they are no longer any use and are a burden to family. It is important to take these expressions very seriously. They do not necessarily mean that individuals are suffering from a major depression that needs to be treated with medication, but they are expressing a strong feeling that reflects dissatisfaction with themselves and their current situation. While many caregivers might be inclined to agree with the sentiments being expressed, to do so without offering anything else may not be very helpful and may merely increase the feeling of afflicted individuals that they really should be dead at this point. Instead, the caregiver should take the position that while these feelings of frustration and despair are very understandable, everyone needs to do all they can to improve the situation as it is now, until it is the right time to die. As noted, many people with Alzheimer's disease who are depressed feel useless, whether or not they are able to express it. Therefore, finding a way to help the person feel a sense of usefulness can be extremely therapeutic. Perhaps that involves identifying some useful chores the person is able to complete successfully on a regular basis: sweeping the garage, weeding the garden, dusting the furniture, or drying the dishes, for example. Being responsible for pet care can be a great source of pleasure and a sense of usefulness for someone with Alzheimer's. This could involve feeding and walking the dog, changing the cat's litter box and feeding the cat; and so forth. Some oversight may be needed depending on the degree of cognitive impairment. Having small grandchildren around can be very helpful, as they can often bring much pleasure to the person with Alzheimer's. In addition, it can be emphasized—accurately—how important it is for the grandchildren to have a chance to spend time with their grandfather or grandmother. The family should encourage the person with Alzheimer's to think of some achievable change in their current situation that might make them feel better. This may uncover some very specific concerns that the person has that could be addressed.

The other common complaint of depressed people with Alzheimer's disease is that they feel like a burden to the family. Nearly all people with Alzheimer's disease express this at one time or another, but when it becomes a major concern for the afflicted person, it needs to be addressed. Most family members will deny that the person with Alzheimer's disease is a burden, but that may not be true, and the affected individual may be astute enough to realize that. While it is important not to blame the Alzheimer's family for the fact that the person feels like a burden, it may be useful for the clinician to explore with family members how burdened they actually feel, and give them an opportunity to both vent about those aspects of the situation that cannot be changed and to problem solve areas where caregiving could be modified to lessen the sense of burden. Some family members who are not happy with having to care for a family member with Alzheimer's may seem to want the afflicted person to realize how burdened they feel, to get the person with Alzheimer's disease to express more gratitude. These are important issues for the clinician to uncover and discuss. It is very understandable that family members may wish their loved one would be more overtly grateful for the care and assistance they are receiving. Indeed, some persons with Alzheimer's are quite verbal about their gratitude and this is enormously helpful for the caregiver. But, unfortunately, many people with the disease are not able to recognize the degree of care and assistance being provided and are not able to express much gratitude for it. Venting one's frustration and wishes with the clinician is far better than expressing this with the person with Alzheimer's, as it will only serve to cause tension and increase the sense of guilt and burden felt by the afflicted person, rather than prompt any spontaneous expressions of gratitude. If the family does feel excessively burdened, they need to consider other ways of providing care, such as involving other family members more, if possible, having more paid caregiver time, or utilizing an adult day program. The critical topic of caregiver burden is discussed in Chapter 8.

When the person with Alzheimer's expresses feeling like a burden, it might be useful for the clinician to help family members to get the person with the disease to see this differently. The family member should remind the afflicted loved one that, in reality, she is giving the family a gift by allowing the family to care for her; that there is equal, if not greater, reward in being able to give care to someone who needs it as there is to receive such care. This type of statement does not deny that there may be burdensome elements in providing care—it would be dishonest to suggest otherwise—but the emphasis is the pleasure and gratitude that the family feels in being able to provide this care. This may be especially the case if the primary caregiver is an adult child of the afflicted individual; then the care provided is merely a reciprocation of care he received earlier in life. This approach can often be helpful in reducing the discomfort and guilt the person with Alzheimer's feels about needing care. But because of the memory impairment, these comments may need to be made repeatedly.

Of course, there needs to be some kernel of truth in this; if all the caregiver feels is anger and resentment for having to take care of the person with Alzheimer's, it would be quite disingenuous to say otherwise, and the person with Alzheimer's would likely sense that the caregiver was not being honest, anyway. The clinician can help family caregivers get in touch with that part of themselves that does actually feel gratified by being a caregiver. This is an important realization for a caregiver to have, as it is often easier to focus only on the negatives. But seeing that caregiving is, in many ways, beneficial to the caregiver as well as to the person receiving care can be an enormously valuable insight.

What about antidepressant medication for the depressed person with Alzheimer's disease? Certainly not every person with Alzheimer's who is sad about the situation requires medication, and medications should never be used simply as an alternative to trying to understand the emotional distress of the person with the disease, and trying to address it psychologically. But when necessary, antidepressants can be extremely helpful for people with Alzheimer's disease who suffer from depression. What are some of the symptoms that might make antidepressant therapy advisable?

- **Severity of the mood disturbance.** One of the factors that should lead to the use of antidepressants is simply the severity of the low mood. Clearly this involves a subjective judgment, but it stands to reason that an individual who is more severely depressed may more urgently need medication than someone whose distress is more mild.
- **Pervasiveness.** The extent to which the lowered mood is present all the time, or nearly all the time, is an indication of

the need for medication. Someone who may have some very sad moments but also feels some genuine sense of happiness at other times may be less in need of antidepressant medication than someone whose mood never improves spontaneously.

- **Anhedonia**. Closely related to the above factor is the presence or absence of anhedonia, which refers to the inability to experience pleasure. Even very severely demented persons with Alzheimer's disease who are not depressed are able to experience and demonstrate positive, pleasurable feelings. It might be a visit from a grandchild, a meal, or some other activity that genuinely pleases the person who is otherwise quite out of contact. But when someone with Alzheimer's disease (and this is true of nondemented people, as well) is unable to experience pleasure in anything, or unable to look forward with pleasure to any future events, then there is almost certainly a significant degree of depression present that probably needs medication to improve. Of course these considerations do not apply to someone who has just suffered a significant loss or is in acute pain from an injury or medical condition. But absent those factors, the presence of anhedonia is almost always a sign of major depression.

- **Irritability.** Some people have been irritable their whole lives, of course; but people with Alzheimer's disease who become significantly irritable may have an underlying depression that will respond well to antidepressant medications. Irritability is one of the more common symptoms of depression in persons with dementia, and it can, of course, make caregiving significantly more difficult than otherwise.

- **Significant loss of appetite or weight loss.** It is common for persons with Alzheimer's disease to lose a few pounds a year; but if weight loss is more rapid than that and appears to be due to loss of appetite, the cause may be depression, and antidepressant medications (particularly certain ones that can increase appetite) can be quite helpful. In very late-stage patients, weight loss may be significant, due to a loss of ability to swallow, and this is often an event that heralds the end of life. This late-stage weight loss is probably not responsive to antidepressants.

- **Frequent crying.** Some people believe that frequent crying is normal for people with Alzheimer's disease. This is certainly not the case, any more so than for people who do not have Alzheimer's disease. While some emotional lability is common in the moderate and later stages of the disease, frequent crying certainly needs to be addressed and may be a symptom that will respond to antidepressant medications.

- **Diurnal mood variation.** Although it is not seen in all cases of depression, some people with major depression have a diurnal pattern of feeling worst in the morning and progressively less depressed as the day goes on, so that by nighttime the mood is much better. But by the next morning, immediately upon awakening, individuals again feel at their worst. Depending on the severity of the depression, mood may not begin to improve until afternoon or early evening, but the pattern repeats itself every day, seven days a week. When this symptom is present, the individual is likely to need antidepressant medication to improve.

- **Rapid functional decline.** While Alzheimer's is a progressive disease in which cognitive and functional symptoms gradually worsen (with or without medication), when decline in cognition or function occurs more rapidly than one would expect on the basis of the disease alone, one of the most common causes is depression. When there is a concern about decline that is more rapid than expected, there should be a thorough evaluation by the treating physician. In the absence of physical causes, it may be that the hastened decline is due to depression. Usually there are other signs of the mood disorder as well, but these can be difficult to discern at times. Treating depression—often with medication—may help stabilize the swift descent and possibly even improve functioning, at least to some degree.

Antidepressant medications are discussed in the appendix.

HANDLING DISINHIBITED OR SOCIALLY INAPPROPRIATE BEHAVIORS

Some degree of disinhibition occurs in most persons with Alzheimer's disease. Loss of judgment and impulse control can lead to a variety of very difficult, inappropriate behaviors.

A slight degree of disinhibition in a person with Alzheimer's who was previously rigid, proper, and humorless can be a welcome development for the family. The person is more talkative, more affectionate, less moralistic perhaps—more fun to be around in some ways. Often, however, the disinhibition does not stop with simply letting one's hair down a little bit, but goes on to create other difficulties.

Symptoms of disinhibition can include relatively minor actions such as leaving the bathroom door open when using the toilet or walking around in an inappropriate state of undress. Other examples are very poor table manners (e.g., spitting food out on the table or the floor); making off-color remarks or swearing when this was not part of the individual's previous style, excessive friendliness with strangers, making lewd remarks, or engaging in sexually inappropriate behaviors.

Individuals with Alzheimer's disease may have no idea that what they are doing is inappropriate, or may understand that caregivers are upset by it, but they do not seem concerned about it, or may even seem amused by the caregiver's reaction. They may offer flimsy excuses, showing no genuine remorse whatsoever. At times, disinhibited behaviors may appear to be premeditated and completely willful, although that is generally an inaccurate and unhelpful view of the situation.

The clinician can play a critical role in helping the caregiver to realize that it is not the person but an unpleasant aspect of the illness that is to blame for these symptoms. The person has not become evil or morally corrupt; these are common symptoms of Alzheimer's disease that can occur in the most morally upstanding, virtuous individuals. The hardest task for the caregiver may be to avoid feeling morally offended or mortified by the behavior. Using firm redirection, distraction, and humor, and avoiding situations in which the symptoms are likely to occur (e.g., by having a male aide if the afflicted individual tends to make sexual overtures to females who assist with care) are all useful. It does no good to ask people not to engage in a certain behavior because it is wrong; if they were capable of that level of understanding or concern, it would not be happening in the first place. It is not a moral issue; it is a brain damage issue.

It is important to control disinhibited, socially inappropriate behaviors not only because of the very negative impact they can have on others, but because of how they cause others to view the person with Alzheimer's, and because such behaviors compromise the person's dignity. When the individual with Alzheimer's disease is no longer able to be concerned about dignity, it becomes the task of the Alzheimer's family to try to maintain and protect it.

Medications may or may not be helpful in dealing with disinhibited behaviors, but because of how disturbing they are, a consultation with the prescribing physician is usually in order. Medications for disinhibition are discussed in the appendix.

MANAGING HALLUCINATIONS

Hallucinations are less common than delusions but do occur in about one quarter of people with Alzheimer's disease. Most often, they are visual (seeing things that are not there), but they can also be auditory (hearing things), tactile (having a physical sensation of something on the skin or in the body), olfactory (smell), or gustatory (taste).

Hallucinations occur in all forms of dementia and may be more common in Lewy body dementia and in Parkinson's dementia than in Alzheimer's disease.

As with delusions, hallucinations are considered a psychotic symptom, but that does not automatically mean that someone should receive antipsychotic medications. Only if the hallucinations are distressing or interfere with function should medication treatment be considered.

At times, the development of hallucinations in someone with Alzheimer's disease is an indication of an underlying acute medical illness (such as a urinary tract infection) that may not be terribly serious by itself but is causing the individual to become delirious. Visual hallucinations are common in delirium.

Possibly the most common hallucination in people with Alzheimer's disease is seeing people in the house. Most often this occurs in the evening or at night after going to bed but before going to sleep, or upon awakening during the night for some reason, such as to go to the bathroom. Hallucinated people almost never speak. The same images may return every day, or a variety of images may be seen. Sometimes they are bizarre, but they may be quite ordinary. Visual hallucinations of animals often occur, as well; these may be ordinary or exotic, such as elephants, giraffes, and so forth.

Persons who are hallucinating are absolutely convinced about the reality of the images, at least initially. If they continue for some time, people may develop awareness that some of them are figments of the imagination but often will insist that at least some of the hallucinations are real. At other times, individuals are completely confused about whether or not the experiences have actually occurred or are simply mental phenomena.

As with delusions, it does no good for the caregiver or other family member to argue about whether or not the hallucinated people are really there. It is best to say something like, "No, I don't see them, but I understand that you do." It is not a good idea for family members to agree that they also see them. If the person does openly question whether the caregiver believes the hallucinations are real, that might be a good opportunity to say, "I don't think they are there, but I know you do; I think maybe it's your mind playing tricks on you" and to focus on the emotional response to the experience—for example, how confusing or upsetting it is, rather than the reality or unreality of the experience itself.

As noted, antipsychotic medications can sometimes be helpful in eliminating hallucinations or reducing their frequency and severity, but, given the side effects of these medications, they should only be used if the hallucinations are quite distressing to the individual, or interfering with functioning (e.g., the person will not go to sleep to make sure the imagined people do not enter the room during the night). Medications for hallucinations are discussed in the appendix.

COPING WITH IRRITABILITY

Irritability is a common symptom of depression in persons with Alzheimer's disease. It can also reflect an underlying paranoid trend. The clinician should try to help the caregiver not take the irritability personally (even though it may be largely or exclusively directed at the primary caregiver). Responding with gentle humor can often be helpful and may help defuse the situation.

Occasionally, persons with Alzheimer's disease become irritable in response to a caregiver's irritability, or caregiver fatigue; it may be appropriate for the clinician to explore whether or not the afflicted individual's irritability could be a response to a change in the family member's behavior or attitude. Once again, it is important for the clinician not to assume that new irritability in the person with Alzheimer's disease is somehow the fault of the caregiver, but merely to use this opportunity to carefully review how the family member is coping with the task. Some family members will complain that the person with Alzheimer's seems to be pleasant with everyone but the primary caregiver and are upset with the unfairness of this, or wonder what they are doing wrong. It can be helpful for the clinician to point out that it is because the afflicted individual feels safest with the primary caregiver that he or she is able to express frustration in this manner. A caregiver who can genuinely not take it personally may be better able to help uncover whether or not the irritable individual is depressed, or if some aspects of the situation are indeed irritating and could perhaps be changed. When irritability is marked, and particularly when it is not a long-standing personality trait of the individual with Alzheimer's, it may be worthwhile to consider antidepressant medication, which can often be quite helpful (see appendix).

MANAGING SLEEP DIFFICULTIES

A variety of sleep problems commonly occur in Alzheimer's disease.

Excessive Sleep

Excessive sleeping is probably the most common sleep disorder in persons with Alzheimer's disease. The individual seems to need an inordinate amount of sleep at night or frequently naps during the day. This symptom may reflect underlying apathy; when left to their own devices, people with apathy do very little and are prone to doze, no matter how much sleep they are routinely getting. If this is the case, then such a person may benefit from more planned activities. The clinician can also work with family members to help them accept the increased need for sleep as a consequence of the illness and encourage them not make inordinate efforts to have the person sleep less. In so doing, the clinician needs to explore why this behavior is upsetting or unacceptable to the family members.

At other times, people with Alzheimer's disease may sleep excessively as a way to withdraw from interactions or implicit demands for functioning and cognitive engagement that they are no longer capable of performing.

Persons who are sleepy during the day despite having adequate amounts of sleep at night may be experiencing side effects of medications that can cause somnolence as a side effect.

Finally, persons with Alzheimer's who sleep excessively during the day may have another sleep disorder, such as sleep apnea. This is to be suspected if there is loud snoring at night, although the actual diagnosis of sleep apnea usually needs to be made by a sleep specialist. It is important to pursue if there are suspicions of sleep apnea, as this condition can lead to worsened cognitive abilities, as well as other medical complications.

Disrupted Sleep

Disrupted sleep includes awakening at night, thinking it is time to get up. It also includes multiple awakenings during the night, other than for the bathroom, with staying up and wandering about the house, often in a very confused state. This can be due to the disruption of the sleep-wake cycle that can occur as part of Alzheimer's disease but could also reflect a significant degree of anxiety. People with a reversed sleep-wake cycle have a tendency to be up a great deal of the night and to sleep during the day.

It may help to limit (but not totally eliminate) daytime napping, particularly naps in the afternoon and certainly naps after supper, if it is difficult for the person with Alzheimer's disease to fall asleep or stay asleep at night. It is also important to ensure that there is adequate activity during the day, and some opportunity for walking or other exercise, commensurate with physical health. Getting outside every day, weather permitting, can be a good routine to develop, one that will help with a variety of matters including nighttime sleep.

If someone tends to get up during the night and wander around the house, and particularly if there is any likelihood of going outside during the night, it may be useful to have alarms on the doors or other devices to make it harder for the individual to leave the house unsupervised without awakening the caregiver.

People with Alzheimer's disease who are up frequently at night can be a very severe drain on the caregiver, particularly if the caregiver is an adult child or younger spouse who goes to work during the day. Helping the caregiver sleep through the night may be reason enough to consider medications to help the afflicted individual sleep, in addition to dealing with the distress the person with Alzheimer's may be experiencing due to sleeplessness. Medications for sleep are discussed in the appendix.

MANAGING SUNDOWNING

Sundowning refers to an increase in confusion or agitation, or other change in behavior, beginning anytime in the second half of the day. It may take the form of pacing, asking repeatedly to go home, general restlessness, irritability, or frank agitation. It may present merely as increased disorientation, forgetfulness, difficulty with tasks that could be performed earlier in the day, or other manifestations of greater cognitive impairment. While there are a number of theories as to why sundowning occurs, it probably has nothing to do with the actual setting of the sun but has that name because the symptoms typically begin in the late afternoon or early evening. It can be very helpful for the clinician to explain sundowning to a family that is confused and troubled by the change in their loved one every afternoon.

The name may not be ideal for a number of reasons, including that it tends to trivialize what can be a very difficult behavior, but it is commonly used. It is a common phenomenon in persons at home, in the hospital, and in long-term care facilities. For many persons, the increase in confusion or other behaviors is noticeable but relatively mild and does not require any special interventions. For others, dramatic changes occur in the later part of every day, which may need some type of intervention to help the individual and the family cope.

Varying hormonal levels during the course of the day, as well as fatigue, hunger, lack of sufficient sleep or exercise, and possibly other factors may contribute to this late-day syndrome. The fatigue of the caregiver late in the day is also a factor that may make interactions more challenging at those times.

Nonpharmacological interventions should include seeing that the individual gets adequate sleep at night and has some daily exercise, ideally outdoors if weather permits. It may be helpful to have a small snack in midafternoon if hunger seems to contribute to the onset of the symptoms. It is also a good idea to avoid cognitively or emotionally demanding activities late in the day, if at all possible. The late afternoon hours may be an excellent time to have a comforting sensory activity, such as a walk, a car ride, listening to music, or having a small snack or a massage. Medication for sundowning is discussed in the appendix.

CHAPTER 8

Caregiver Stress

One of the most difficult things about Alzheimer's disease is the great amount of time that individuals and their families are affected. The duration of the illness, from the time of diagnosis to the time of death, is usually between 5 and 15 years. In addition, symptoms have usually been present for several years prior to the diagnosis. Caregiving becomes more and more time consuming, and in many ways more difficult, as the disease progresses. Clearly, the family must make a long-term commitment to this task. A major part of one's commitment needs to be to care for oneself and the rest of the family during the process. This is essential not only for the obvious reason that the Alzheimer's family members themselves deserve it, but also for a more practical one: maintaining one's own health and well-being and that of the family during the long caregiving journey makes it possible to continue caregiving for a longer period of time. If caregivers become so stressed that they become ill, or reach a point emotionally of being unable to do the job any longer, and other family members cannot take over fully, the person with the disease may need to go into long-term residential care as a result. In fact, one of the main reasons for premature placement in a nursing home is that, for a variety of reasons, caregiver stress becomes so great that the caregiver can no longer cope and needs to give up the task. This can occur for any number of reasons, including the following:

- Not getting sufficient assistance from others
- Setting one's standards so high that they cannot possibly be met
- Caring for a person whose behaviors are particularly challenging
- Having a relationship with the afflicted person that was difficult or unrewarding even before the illness

This is not to say that every nursing home placement represents a failure on the part of the Alzheimer's family—far from it. Most caregivers and families do a fine job of caring for their loved one at home, but sooner or later the increasing demands overwhelm even the best, most devoted caregivers. Nor is it to say that placement in a nursing facility is necessarily a poor outcome. Most people with Alzheimer's disease do, in fact, end up in nursing home care by late in the illness, and those in good facilities often have a very reasonable quality of life from that point forward. However, placement is usually something that most people and families would like to avoid or delay as long as possible. Coping well with the stress of caregiving helps achieve this goal. Nursing home placement is discussed in greater detail in Chapter 9.

RECOGNIZING THE SIGNS OF CAREGIVER STRESS

Even in families that are loving and mutually supportive, who share the caregiving duties and have prepared themselves well for the task, there will be times when the burdens of caring for the person Alzheimer's disease become very challenging, indeed. Caregiver stress can take many forms. Some of the common symptoms of caregiver stress include the following:

- Being obsessively preoccupied with thoughts about the afflicted person
- Excessive anger, particularly directed at the person with Alzheimer's

- Feeling overwhelmed with the tasks of caregiving
- Feeling a loss of control over one's own life
- Disengagement from social activities and other interests
- Feeling exhausted all the time, but having difficulty sleeping
- Symptoms of depression
- Being preoccupied with guilt over not doing enough for the person with Alzheimer's
- Excessive worry, anxiety, or irritability

In addition, caregivers under significant stress have more medical problems than do similarly aged individuals who are not caregivers but may not go to the doctor often enough because their concerns are focused exclusively on the person with Alzheimer's. This puts their health in jeopardy.

SPECIFIC CAUSES OF STRESS IN THE ALZHEIMER'S FAMILY

The causes of stress are myriad and obvious, to a great degree. But there are some factors that deserve mentioning.

- **Grief over the gradual loss of a loved one.** This may be the most significant stressor on any caregiver. Managing the ongoing grief of losing a spouse or a parent to Alzheimer's is perhaps the greatest challenge for the members of the Alzheimer's family. It is also the most important area for clinicians to address and work with throughout their time with the Alzheimer's family. Grief is discussed in detail in Chapter 10.
- **"The 36-hour day."** Mace and Rabins (2006) popularized the concept of the 36-hour day in their excellent book of the same name. This refers to the notion that, from the caregiver's perspective, there is no time available for anything other than caring for the person with Alzheimer's disease. Even if this is not factually true, the feeling of being totally taken over by the demands of caregiving is very real indeed, and is a significant cause of caregiver stress.
- **Poor premorbid relationships.** Perhaps it is obvious that car-

ing for someone toward whom one feels a deep sense of love and commitment is easier than caring for someone with whom there has been a conflicted, distant, or tempestuous relationship throughout the marriage. Similarly, if the caregiver is an adult child, it is certainly easier to devote oneself to someone who has been a wonderful parent in every respect and has been deeply and unambivalently loved by the adult child. But when the parent-child relationship has been stormy, or abusive, many adult children will opt out of being involved as caregivers at all. Those that do take on the task often do so out of a feeling of guilt, a desire to help the other parent, or a hope that they can be a better caregiver to their parent than the parent was to them. The adult child hopes that doing so will ameliorate some of the long-standing problems that have plagued the relationship but may have previously been handled simply by avoidance. Indeed, it is possible that a troubled marital or parent-child relationship can be improved during Alzheimer's disease, which is deeply gratifying when it does occur. But even in those situations, and especially when there is no significant improvement in the relationship, taking care of someone about whom one has a great deal of ambivalence is enormously stressful. There is, to start, simply less desire to go out of one's way for the individual who perhaps never was kind in the first place. Interactions tend to be fraught with difficult emotions. The caregiver often has difficulty controlling angry and resentful feelings toward the individual. If these are not explored and vented with the clinician, they may come out in indirect ways such as focusing on the cognitive and functional impairments of the person with Alzheimer's. If the person who now has Alzheimer's was always critical of the spouse, this negative mode of interacting will usually continue, without the periodic expressions of gratitude that all caregivers need to continue to perform the job with any degree of equanimity. If this is the atmosphere between the person with Alzheimer's and the caregiver and other family members, it is important for the family to express their dissatisfaction with the situation to the clinician but not necessarily to the person with Alzheimer's. However, it is important to be clear about what is needed from the person with Alzheimer's (e.g., "Stop criticizing everything I do"). This may bring about some at least temporary improvement in the interactions, although given the memory impairment and long-established patterns of interacting, it may not last, unfortunately. Nevertheless, it can be helpful to caregivers to express their feelings in this way, even if the external situation does not really change very much.

- **Stress from mood and behavioral symptoms.** Mood and behavioral symptoms in the person with Alzheimer's disease contribute significantly to the sense of stress and burden felt by the Alzheimer's family, particularly the primary caregiver. All of the common behavioral symptoms in Alzheimer's disease (see Chapter 7) can be a source of significant stress for the family. As noted earlier, it can be helpful for the family to try to determine identifiable precipitants for particular behaviors, or specific circumstances that seem to make the problems worse or better. Certainly the clinician can assist in this exploration by helping to review the sequence of events that seemed to lead to an episode of difficult behavior. This may help improve the situation and also give the family members some sense of control, which is critical in lessening the tension that is inevitable with these behaviors. Feeling victimized by behavioral symptoms and feeling that nothing can be done about it will substantially increase stress. In reviewing the behavioral events, the clinician may want to suggest a visit with the prescribing physician; medication may be helpful in controlling the symptoms (see appendix).

CAREGIVER BURNOUT

Caregiver burnout refers to an extreme degree of caregiver stress that has usually been building for a considerable period of time. It often appears that the caregiver may be nearing the end of his or her ability to continue in the role. When a caregiver appears to be reaching this point, urgent action is required, as the safety and well-being of both the caregiver and the person with Alzheimer's may be in jeopardy.

Sometimes the first awareness anyone has of caregiver burnout is when the caregiver announces that he or she can simply no longer continue caregiving any longer. When it comes as a surprise, it usually means that the family was not paying sufficient attention (which may also have contributed to the burnout) because there are usually hints of this coming long before it actually happens. The clinician may need to decide whether to try to help the caregiver continue in the role longer or to immediately assist in finding alternate arrangements for the person with Alzheimer's. Often, simply asking the caregiver will determine the answer to that question, although the clinician cannot be certain when the caregiver is overwrought about the situation. When the goal seems to be to help the caregiver feel better enough to continue caregiving, at least for some period of time, it may be helpful to attempt to find out if there were particular incidents that brought about the decision to give up as a caregiver. If such incidents are uncovered, some effort to address those specific incidents may be worthwhile. For example, the individual with Alzheimer's disease may have developed diarrhea, possibly due to antidementia medications, and because of the diarrhea is no longer continent of bowel. Many caregivers draw the line at having to clean up incontinent stool. If this is the case, a consultation with the physician may lead to treatment of diarrhea, with a result that the incontinence is solved, and the caregiver is willing to go on.

In other cases, the caregiver may not be able to define any particular incidents that have caused the feeling of being unable to continue. It may simply be that the accumulation of cognitive difficulties, functional problems, and behavioral issues has led to that point. It is always useful to ask if there is anything that would lead caregivers to continue longer. If they are able to identify anything, within reason, that would make a difference, all effort should be made to see if the desired change could be effected. But frequently, caregivers will already have their minds made up before they announce that they can no longer continue to provide care, and it is important to heed this warning. Not doing so could put the person with Alzheimer's disease at risk.

A common concomitant of burnout is severe depression in the caregiver, with difficulty functioning in both caregiving tasks and noncaregiving aspects of life. The caregiver may be doing what is needed, barely, to provide necessary care for the person with Alzheimer's but spends no other time or energy interacting with him or her, and spends much of the time in bed or sitting and functioning only minimally.

Another common and worrisome sign of caregiver burnout can be anger that is expressed with increasing frequency at the afflicted person, in destructive ways. The caregiver may be significantly sleep deprived, not only because the person with Alzheimer's is up and down frequently at night but because the caregiver may have difficulty falling or staying asleep. Early morning awakening, before it is time to get up, and being unable to return to sleep is an important symptom of depression. If suicidal feelings are present, an emergency psychiatric evaluation is necessary.

As caregivers reach the burnout stage, the risk of neglect or abuse of the person with Alzheimer's disease increases. Of course, neglect or abuse can occur at any time, but whenever it happens, a major change in the arrangements must occur immediately.

Abuse by the caregiver can take many forms. Physical violence toward the individual is of course the most concerning issue, but more subtle forms of physical abuse include, for example, rough handling when assisting the person with bathing or dressing. If someone needs help getting up from the toilet, for example, leaving him there an unnecessarily long time can be viewed as a type of physical abuse, because of the discomfort caused.

Verbal abuse includes yelling and cursing at the individual but can also include insulting or demeaning comments that intentionally focus on the individual's cognitive or functional problems rather than on those areas of preserved abilities. More subtle forms of verbal abuse might be expressed not so much in the words that are said to the afflicted individual as in the tone that is used.

One would not expect most burned-out caregivers to report these indicators of abuse. If they are aware of them, there is likely a great deal of shame and embarrassment about their behavior. But in many cases, caregivers may not have insight into their abusiveness. It is therefore important for the clinician to ask caregivers to recount specific interactions with the afflicted person, in detail, when there are any concerns of this kind. The goal is to help caregivers come to recognize that their interactions with the afflicted person have been inappropriate and to begin to discuss how best to handle this crisis. However, if caregivers are not able to reach this awareness themselves, it is still necessary for the clinician to make explicit that the behaviors described are abusive and need to stop. It may be necessary for the clinician to call in other members of the family to assist with this crisis.

The uncovering of abuse is an immediate call for more help for the caregiver, whether or not other actions are taken. The help may be greater assistance from other family members, although if relatives are nearby and the situation has reached this point, it may mean that these family members are not sufficiently engaged, and an urgent family session should be held so the clinician can emphasize the seriousness of the situation and find out what help they can offer. If no other family members are available, it may be necessary to hire private caregivers to come in, if this is possible financially. It also may mean it is time to actively consider nursing home placement.

Caregiver neglect is an equally serious problem. It can be harder to determine, except in extreme cases, such as when a person with Alzheimer's who needs considerable assistance is left alone for many hours or overnight, or is left in a car for several hours while the caregiver goes shopping. Neglect can be more subtle as well. It may be that all of a person's basic needs are met but he or she is essentially ignored the rest of the time. Again, the caregiver may not report these behaviors, but thorough questioning may uncover evidence of more subtle neglect. This is why it is always helpful for the clinician to meet with other members of the family when there are any concerns about abuse or neglect. Other family members may not be fully accurate in their description of the situation, either, but the additional point of view is always valuable in situations like this.

REPORTING THE ABUSIVE OR NEGLECTFUL CAREGIVER

Making the decision to report the stressed caregiver who is abusing or neglecting the person with Alzheimer's disease is very difficult and should not be taken lightly; however, if the clinician has a serious concern that the safety and well-being of the person with Alzheimer's disease is in jeopardy, it is essential that the clinician take this action. While it may feel like the clinician is violating the caregiver's trust, the safety of the person with Alzheimer's disease overrides that concern. Furthermore, most states have laws that require the reporting of elder abuse or neglect, just as they require the reporting of child abuse. In addition, reporting someone may be a way of getting additional help for the caregiver at home. When the clinician decides to report a caregiver, he or she should inform the caregiver of this, unless it is felt that doing so would put the person with Alzheimer's disease in imminent danger. Otherwise, the clinician should emphasize that the goal of reporting is not to punish the caregiver in any way but to protect the person with Alzheimer's and to get immediate assistance with what is obviously a very difficult situation. It is also appropriate to notify the physician of the concern and the action being taken.

When the clinician has to go to the extreme of reporting a caregiver, it means that a major change in the caregiving arrangements needs to occur immediately. Perhaps the person with Alzheimer's disease can live with a different relative, at least temporarily while arrangements are being made for more professional caregivers to be hired. It may also mean that nursing home placement is now necessary.

CHAPTER 9

Long-Term Care

As the disease goes on over several years, and the individual progressively declines cognitively and functionally, he or she generally becomes increasingly difficult to manage at home, and the family often begins to consider placement in a long-term care facility. This usually occurs when the patient is on the more impaired end of the moderate stage of dementia and is approaching the severe stage. Typical signs and symptoms in this late moderate stage of the disease include the following:

- Inability to perform any instrumental activities of daily living
- Some difficulty basic activities of daily living—dressing, toileting, maintaining hygiene, and eating independently
- Unsteady ambulation, with a history of falling
- Reluctance or frequent refusal to bathe
- Disorientation
- Very poor to nonexistent short-term memory
- Significant aphasia; inabilty to carry on a meaningful conversation
- Agnosias are present: considerable difficulty recognizing people who should be familiar, and some difficulty reliably recognizing close family members

Behavioral symptoms are common at this point and may include the following:

- Sleep disturbances with wandering around the house at night, or significant difficulties with sleeping
- Agitation at times of care
- Delusional ideation; occasional hallucinations
- Significant mood dysregulation with periods of significant depression, marked irritability, or overt aggressiveness

Individuals at this point in the disease generally need to have someone with them, or nearby in the house, all the time. If they had previously lived alone, they are no longer by themselves or certainly should not be. If they do not live with family, they need to have someone else living with them full-time to ensure safety.

Some families will opt to provide maximal care at home, either by family members or by a combination of family and paid helpers. Having adequate help at home can significantly delay placement in a long-term care facility. Some people with Alzheimer's disease are able to remain at home until the end of their lives, if there are sufficient resources to provide full-time care at home. Full-time paid care at home costs about the same as nursing home care. For most families, professional home care providers must be paid primarily out of pocket as insurance rarely assists with this.

For many families, however, keeping the person with Alzheimer's disease at home until the end of life is simply not possible or even desirable. It is certainly not a sign of weakness or failure on the part of a family to need to place a loved one in long-term care. By this point in the illness, the ravages of the disease have usually overtaken the ability of even the best caregiving families to continue to manage the individual at home. More often than not, placement is something the family has been considering for months, if not longer. However, active consideration and planning often get put off for a considerable period of time, because of the enormous guilt caused by the idea of placement. Some families have unwisely promised they would never put the afflicted person in a care facility, and as placement looks more and more necessary, they are tremendously conflicted about the situation. The clinician should strongly advise family members never to make that promise, but it may already have been made before the first visit to the clinician. At an earlier stage of the illness, the family may genuinely have felt that they could manage whatever would develop and were committed to keeping the loved one at home, as a matter of loyalty and love for the person with Alzheimer's. This is especially the case when family members or perhaps the afflicted individual have unpleasant recollections of a relative languishing in a nursing home in the past. Indeed, nursing home care was quite different a generation ago, with patients often overmedicated, restrained, and largely ignored, or worse. Because of this poor treatment, the Nursing Home Reform Act of 1987 was passed by Congress and went into effect in 1990. This regulation established standards of quality for nursing home care nationwide. The law was tied to the Omnibus Budget Reconciliation Act (OBRA) of 1987, and so these nursing home regulations are often referred to today as the OBRA laws. This reform act, and its enforcement through annual surveys of nursing homes, has meant a substantial improvement in the quality of care throughout the nursing home industry.

At times, individuals who could be (and perhaps should be) placed in a care facility remain at home for financial reasons. The cost of long-term institutional care is considerable. Families must pay out of pocket, unless they have long-term care insurance, which most do not. Once they have spent down their assets very significantly, the individual becomes eligible for Medicaid, but this can certainly devastate the family savings.

As noted in Chapter 8, if the primary caregiver reaches a stage of burnout or becomes abusive or neglectful, long-term care placement may become an urgent matter. It can also occur because of illness or even death of the primary caregiver or some other unexpected, sudden change in the caregiving situation that makes it no longer possible to provide sufficient care at home. But most often, the move to placement occurs gradually and families have time to examine the options.

Leaving aside financial considerations, guilt, and promises perhaps made to the person with the disease, when should someone go into a long-term care facility? There is no correct time for placement. In many cases, when someone is admitted to a care facility for long-term care, a review of the situation suggests that placement could have—and perhaps should have—occurred many months earlier. The primary factor delaying it is almost always caregiver guilt.

Making a decision about placement involves a complex set of factors having to do with the needs of the person with Alzheimer's, the caregiver's status, and the availability of alternative resources. However, a number of considerations, when present, indicate a definite need for some sort of placement:

- The physical or mental health of the caregiver has become seriously jeopardized by the burdens of caregiving.
- The person with Alzheimer's disease wanders out of the house unsafely, and measures to control this have been unsuccessful.
- Behavioral symptoms have become unmanageable in the home setting.
- There is a need for more physical care than can be provided by available caregivers in the home.
- There are financial or practical reasons why full-time, around-the-clock care cannot be provided at home—or the person with Alzheimer's disease will not accept it.
- The person with dementia no longer recognizes home or does not recognize the primary caregiver.

This final point bears further explanation: people who do not recognize their home are at high risk to wander, with the vain hope of finding home or somewhere that seems familiar. Being in an environment or with caregivers whom they do not recognize can be quite upsetting and can lead to aggressive outbursts, even when they have not occurred before. It is also the case that family members often feel that they are more willing to place a loved one who always wanted to remain at home when that loved one no longer recognizes home.

TYPES OF LONG-TERM CARE FACILITIES

One of the first considerations in thinking about long-term care is the type of facility. There is some variability from one commu-

nity or region to another, but in general the four main types of care
facilities which are appropriate for the person with Alzheimer's
disease are as follows:

1. Board and care homes
2. Assisted living facilities
3. Nursing homes
4. Continuing care retirement communities

Board and Care Homes

Small facilities of less than 12 residents, often board and care
homes have been converted from large older houses. They offer
meals, medication supervision, assistance with activities of daily
living, and some activities, but generally there is not a nurse on
premises all the time, as is the case in other facilities (see below).
Because they are small, they do not have an institutional feel and
can be very homelike. Some facilities tend not to take people with
Alzheimer's disease or other dementias, while others may special-
ize in that type of care. Because of the small size, they have relatively minimal services and are suitable for persons who are on the
milder end of the spectrum of disease, but in need of daily care.
They are usually less expensive than the other facilities listed
below. Their availability and the services provided vary widely in
different communities.

Assisted Living Facilities

Assisted living facilities (ALFs) have multiplied in the last decade or so, as entrepreneurs have recognized the changing demo-
graphics of our society, with increasing numbers of seniors and
fewer adult children able or willing to take them in when they
need help. ALFs vary greatly in terms of services provided. They
are generally larger than board and care homes. Some offer little
more than apartment living with a communal meal once a day.
However, most offer more assistance and tend to care for persons
with greater needs than board and care homes will take. About
25% of ALFs have dementia-specific units, or the entire facility is
designed for persons with Alzheimer's disease or other dementias.

Memory care units usually have a locked door, to be safe for people who would otherwise wander. Memory care units within an assisted living facility have higher staff/resident ratios and ideally have staff members who have been specifically trained to care for persons with Alzheimer's disease. There may be more activities on the memory care units than on the general assisted living units, and the activities tend to be geared more toward those with cognitive impairment. Memory care units tend to cost more per month—often considerably more—than regular ALF units.

In general, ALFs are less institutional than nursing homes and may be more homelike, pleasant environments. Most rooms are single, except for couples who come to the facility together, compared to the double rooms of most older nursing homes. There is nicer furniture and better food, usually, than nursing homes. Residents in assisted living tend to be less severely demented, even on the memory care units, than in nursing homes, and need less nursing care than those in nursing homes. Overall, there tends to be less behavioral disturbance on assisted living memory units compared to nursing home memory units. Also, there tend to be fewer medically ill, bedbound, or wheelchair-bound patients. In many states, assisted living patients must be able to self-evacuate in case of a fire (meaning they can get out on their own) while that is not the case, certainly, in a nursing home. While many ALFs try to keep their residents until the end of life, others cannot manage the physical care needs of the person with more advanced disease and will then transfer the individual to a nursing home. Also, while in some states ALFs may keep residents once they have exhausted their personal funds and gone onto Medicaid, this is not the case everywhere.

Nursing Homes

Nursing homes are widely variable, of course. Many have units for skilled nursing care; these units are for individuals who have been transferred to the facility from a hospital, for rehabilitation from a stroke or a fractured hip, or any other illness for which the individual no longer needs the services of the acute care hospital but needs rehabilitation to get well enough to be able to go home.

Patients who are transferred into skilled nursing care are covered by Medicare, whereas long-term patients in the nursing home are not. Typical Alzheimer's patients who go to a nursing home are admitted to long-term care, where they may be on a general unit with individuals with various ailments, including dementia, or may be admitted to a nursing home dementia unit. A significant percentage of nursing homes have special care units for persons with Alzheimer's disease and other dementias. These are similar to the memory care units in ALFs in that there is typically limited egress (a locked door), more dementia-specific activities, and sometimes a physical environment that is "dementia friendly." As noted above, residents in the nursing home, particularly those on dementia units, tend to have more advanced disease, and there may be more behavioral problems.

Generally, assisted living tends to be preferred by families, as well as by individuals with dementia, unless they are quite significantly impaired, in which case the particular locale may not be as meaningful to the individual. What matters most at that point (at any point, actually) is not the physical amenities but the kindness and sophistication of the staff and the overall quality of care they are able to provide, given the particular needs of these individuals.

Continuing Care Retirement Communities

Continuing care retirement communities (CCRCs) generally offer the full range of care from independent living in apartments or cottages to assisted living, to nursing home care, often (but not always) with dementia-specific units. One of the great advantages of CCRCs is that they allow individuals and families to "age in place." Generally, people move into a CCRC when they are able to live independently; as time goes on and needs increase, the individual can move, within the facility, to a higher level of care. Of course, going to a CCRC takes advance planning, and many have considerable waiting lists. Most will not accept someone into the facility who needs a dementia care unit at the time of admission.

For the family beginning to consider placement, deciding which of these types of facilities is appropriate is the first step. The clinician can certainly provide guidance in this respect. The type of

facility chosen will likely be determined by the clinical characteristics of the afflicted individual, but financial considerations may
also be relevant. Next, the family must choose a specific facility.
Depending on the area, there may be many choices or only one or
two that are nearby. Generally it is important to choose a facility
that is convenient for family to visit, assuming the nearby facilities
are considered acceptable. A very well-known, high-quality facility an hour away that has openings is not necessarily the right
choice unless the facilities that are closer are of much lower quality.

How does one judge the quality of a facility? It is necessary to
look beyond the marketing materials and the appearance of the
building. It is a good idea to visit, unannounced if possible, and
have a good look at the residents and the staff. Consider these
questions:

- Do the residents seem happy?
- Are residents engaged in activities or conversations with one
  another, or with staff members?
- Are the residents inactive, disconnected from one another
  and from the staff?
- Are residents in the common areas, or are they in their own
  rooms in front of the television?
- Do residents appear clean and well groomed, or are they
  wearing soiled pajamas or clothes and show signs of ne-
  glected grooming?
- Are staff members readily visible?
- Do staff members appear happy, as if they are enjoying their
  work?
- Are the staff members engaged with the residents or only
  talking with each other?
- Do the staff members spend any time interacting with the
  residents when they perform tasks for them (e.g., administering medications, assisting with ADLs)?

If possible, try to find out how long people have worked at the facility (assuming it is not brand new). The best facilities tend to
have staff members who have worked there for a long time. Any
long-term care facility, assisted living, or nursing home will have

young aides who are relatively inexperienced and transient; but is there a core of more experienced staff? Those facilities that tend to keep staff longer are, as a general rule, better places to work, and therefore usually better places in which to reside. And since persons with dementia need sameness and stability, a facility whose staff is constantly changing is probably one to be avoided.

Recommendations from families who have had loved ones in the facility are important; the recommendation of the physician is valuable as well, although physicians tend to have a different view of facilities than people who have actually had a relative living there. Finally, facilities are rated by the state, and these ratings are publicly available on the Internet. Facilities that have had a great number of deficiencies may have systemic problems and possibly should be avoided. On the other hand, a deficiency-free survey is no guarantee that an individual and family will be satisfied with a particular facility. In the end, all of these factors need to be considered, but the final decision in choosing an ALF or nursing home may rest on a general overall impression that a particular place is, or is not, the right place for one's family member.

There may be disagreement in the family about placing someone in a care facility. Frequently, the person objecting strongly to the placement is not involved in the daily care of the afflicted person and really does not understand how overwhelming the task is. It can be useful for the clinician to suggest that the objecting family member spend several days, at least, in the shoes of the primary caregiver. This will often help the family member see what is involved. The final decision about placement must rest with the primary caregiver, but this difficult decision is certainly easier if there is strong and unanimous family support. But if the primary caregiver does not feel capable of doing the job any longer, it may not be in the best interests of the person with Alzheimer's to stay at home. It is not infrequent that adult children are unanimous in their desire for the well parent to place the afflicted spouse in a facility, because of their concern about the negative impact of the disease on the primary caregiver. While the adult children may be very correct in their assessment of the situation, they often do not appreciate the enormous sense of duty that spouses feel to care for their loved one "until the end"; or they may not appreciate the gratification the well spouse is getting from being a caregiver, despite the great burdens being inflicted. These are situations in which it would be very beneficial to have some family meetings with the clinician to discuss what is best for both members of the couple. Once a decision is reached to move the person with Alzheimer's disease to a care setting, it is extremely important that the involved family members be unanimous. This will generally make it easier for the afflicted person to accept the placement. Ambivalence in the family can be sensed, which can make the situation much more difficult for everyone. Also, agreement in the family about the need for placement will help the primary caregiver deal more effectively with guilt about the plan.

It is important for caregivers and families not to view placement in assisted living or a nursing home as an undesirable necessity that occurs simply because care can no longer be managed at home. It is useful, and accurate, to think about the positive benefits a good care facility can offer, over and above what the home environment might provide. Here it is critical to view the situation from the perspective of the impaired individual, not from one's own perspective. It is hard to imagine anyone cognitively intact choosing to live in a memory care unit of an ALF or a nursing home, any more than anyone would choose to develop Alzheimer's disease. But there are important benefits a good care facility can offer the person who is significantly cognitively impaired, including the following:

- Specialized dementia training of the staff
- Availability of care providers 24 hours a day
- Assistance with activities of daily living whenever it is needed
- Medication administration
- An appropriate physical environment designed with the needs of people with dementia in mind
- A daily schedule of activities appropriate for the person with cognitive impairment

- The opportunity for interaction with other individuals who have similar difficulties
- Limited egress

Placing a demented individual in a facility permits the family to step back from the caregiving role and return to the opportunity to enjoy the individual simply from the perspective of being a spouse, an adult child, a grandchild, and so on. It certainly is best for families to have memories of doing enjoyable activities together, or of having simple quiet visits, rather than struggling over dressing, bathing, toileting, and the like. The person with advanced dementia may indeed need a great deal of physical and other caregiving but perhaps needs a spouse, or loving adult daughter or son, even more.

INVOLVING THE PERSON WITH ALZHEIMER'S DISEASE IN THE DECISION FOR PLACEMENT

While it would be ideal if the afflicted individual could fully participate in the placement decision and agree that such a move were necessary, this is rare, unfortunately. By the time people with Alzheimer's disease need to go to a care facility, they have usually lost insight into the severity of the condition and tend to greatly overstate their abilities. They are rarely able to see or appreciate the extent of the care being provided by the spouse and other members of the Alzheimer's family, or feel that whatever is being done could and should continue in the home environment indefinitely. Because people with Alzheimer's disease who have progressed to this stage of illness have significant impairments in judgment and other higher-level cognitive tasks, it may be futile to offer a thoughtful presentation as to why placement has become necessary, from the caregiver's perspective, and why it may be helpful and enjoyable for the afflicted person. Nevertheless, it may be reasonable to try this approach. The nature of the afflicted person's reaction to such a presentation may determine if and when further attempts should be made to use logic and reason in the hopes of persuading the person to agree. When a person with

Alzheimer's completely refuses to go to a care facility, it can be very difficult for the family Even when there is strong refusal, it may be helpful to frequently bring up the idea so that it is (temporarily at least) in the mind of the person with Alzheimer's disease. However, if it simply causes a great deal of agitation, this approach may need to be abandoned.

At times, families decide that it will be easier for all concerned not to bring up the issue of placement with the afflicted individual at all but simply to take the person to the facility one day, ostensibly for lunch or something, and then have the afflicted person remain. Others will say that the person is going into the facility for now or for a short while, perhaps because the caregiver needs to be out of town or unavailable for some other reason, but convey that the placement is only for a brief period, when they know otherwise. Once again, it is important to emphasize that there is no right way to do this very difficult task. The primary caregiver and other family members could benefit from speaking to the clinician to develop a plan for how to make the transition, and to help deal with the enormous feelings of guilt that result.

ACTIVE PLANNING FOR ADMISSION

Once the decision has been made about placement and the facility has been selected, there are a number of steps to take that will help ease the transition. The day of admission should be determined. There should not be a long gap between the decision to admit and the actual admission date, as this may be too difficult for the family to handle emotionally, and the individual with Alzheimer's will likely be affected. Allow only enough time to make the necessary arrangements. First, the local family members who work outside of their homes should arrange to take the day off, if at all possible. They can be very helpful in transporting the individual and providing support for the primary caregiver. They can also help with transporting personal effects from home to the facility and setting up the individual's room so it is as familiar and comfortable as possible.

The physician should be notified, if he or she has not been an active part of the decision making about the timing of placement. He or she will need to complete paperwork for the facility. If this physician is not able to continue as the person's doctor once the admission has occurred, he or she can assist with planning for a transition to a new doctor at the facility. Medication orders will need to be brought or sent to the facility, and it is frequently useful to have additional doses of a "prn" (as needed) calming medication available, should the transition cause the person to become anxious or agitated. When a new patient in the facility urgently needs some medication to calm down is not the time the facility should have to start tracking down the doctor, get an order, and get the medicine from the pharmacy. Some families ask to have their loved one "snowed" (medicated to the point of excessive sedation) prior to admission, and while that extreme should not be necessary, it may be a good idea to administer an extra dose of calming medication prior to traveling to the facility for admission.

ADMISSION DAY

The day of admission to a facility is sometimes described by family members as the worst day of their lives. To some degree that has to do with the individual's negative reactions to the move, but to an even greater degree it has to do with the caregiver's extreme sadness and guilt. The caregiver often suffers more than the person with Alzheimer's disease during the transition to long-term care (and at other times, as well).

The family should ascertain from the facility the best time to bring the person for admission (if they have not already specified this) and then should adhere to it. It is not ideal to admit the person at a time when the staff are tied up with other activities. It is usually not a good idea to admit someone on a Friday, if it can be avoided, because the weekend staff beginning Friday night or Saturday may not be as numerous or as experienced as those present during the week.

Particularly if the person does not understand ahead of time that he or she is being admitted to the facility, it is a good idea not to travel to the facility with lots of suitcases or other items, as this is likely to provoke anxiety. The ideal situation would be to bring the person's belongings and room decorations to the facility in another car. While the person with Alzheimer's and the spouse or other primary caregiver are having lunch or visiting in the day room, other family members could be hard at work unpacking and setting up the room, so that by the time the individual sees the new room for the first time, it looks familiar and inviting and is not cluttered with boxes or suitcases.

Leaving the person with Alzheimer's alone in the facility can be excruciating for family members, but it must be done. It should happen without great fanfare, and without long, tearful goodbyes. It is best if a staff member can be with the afflicted person at that time, to engage the person in an activity that might help distract the individual, at least somewhat, from the family's departure.

THE INITIAL ADJUSTMENT PERIOD

Most facilities will make recommendations about the frequency of visits during the first days and weeks after admission. It is a good idea for family to try to accept these recommendations, as they are usually based on what the staff have found works best with other new admissions. There is a risk that family visits that are too frequent or too lengthy will prevent the person from settling into the facility, learning the routines and the people there, and beginning to make some friends. It may be very hard for family to limit their visits, but this may be, in the long run, best for the loved one.

Telephone calls can be made to the staff, if family members are very concerned about how their loved one is doing, but these should not be excessive, as the staff's first priority is to be with the residents and not on the phone reassuring family members. It is also a good idea to find out the best time to call, and when telephone calls should be avoided (at change of shift or mealtimes, perhaps). When called, staff will commonly say that someone is doing just fine and getting settled in well, but when family visit, they see a very different picture: the person with Alzheimer's is clinging and demands to go home. Indeed, the staff member has likely described the situation accurately; it is only when the family visit that the sentiments about going home are brought to the surface, by the family's very presence. In extreme situations, this may mean that visiting should occur less frequently.

Family members should realize that the initial days or even weeks following admission may be the most difficult for them to endure. It may, or may not, be the most difficult time for the person with Alzheimer's as well, but with the passage of time, the situation nearly always improves. During this time, it would be advisable not to take the person out of the facility, and certainly not to bring the person back home, even for a holiday. Such home visits would only prolong the period of adjustment for the person who has Alzheimer's, and it may be difficult to get the person to agree to go back to the facility after a visit home. If it is clear that the person will not be able to live at home again, then it may be kindest to facilitate the home setting becoming more of a blur until, thanks to the memory loss of Alzheimer's disease, it fades largely or completely from memory. Taking someone home for a visit who strongly wants to be there permanently can be seen as a tease, akin to giving a starving person just one bite of a delicious steak. That one bite will bring no satisfaction, only a greatly increased craving for the food.

Even if the worst of the initial transition period has passed, it is still inadvisable to take the person back home, or even to the neighborhood, because this will stir up a desire to be back home on a permanent basis. However, going out for walks, car rides, or to a local restaurant may be quite reasonable. Visits at the facility are best kept relatively brief—long visits can be quite trying for both sides. It is best if visits can be focused around an activity—doing something rather than simply sitting and talking, as one might do if visiting a cognitively intact friend or relative in the hospital. It has probably been a long time since it was possible to sit and have a lengthy conversation with the individual with the disease, and trying to do that now is unlikely to be effective. It is also good to plan visits at times of day when the individual feels best—perhaps midmorning—and to plan to leave at a time when the person can be distracted by an activity, perhaps a meal or something else that will gain his or her attention. If the person with Alzheimer's repeatedly asks his visitors to bring him home, a firm but kind answer that this is not possible should be given. If the afflicted individual persists in pleading to go home, it may be necessary to terminate the visit at that point, as the situation is only likely to worsen if the caregiver remains and tries to use logic to explain why the person needs to remain at the facility. Some persons with Alzheimer's will attempt to play on family members' guilt to try to get taken home, and it helps if the family member can avoid showing too much guilt about it.

How often should one visit? As before, there is no single correct answer to this question. For most family members, visits should probably occur somewhat less frequently than one is inclined. The frequency of visiting has more to do with the caregiver's needs than those of the person with the disease. After all, most people who are impaired enough to require placement are not likely to be able to tell whether the caregiver visited just yesterday or several days ago. It is common in facilities to see patients complain to family who visit daily that they never see them; and it is also common that family members who are away for a period of a few weeks may return to find that the absence seemed no different for the person than an absence of only a day or two. Thus family members should come as often as they feel the need to, recognizing that the visits are largely for them, even more than for the loved one.

Family members who were not directly involved in the day-to-day care of the person with Alzheimer's at home may have the impression that, now that placement has occurred, the stresses on the primary caregiver are over. That is certainly not the case. The nature of the stress changes, but for most family members it remains significant. Struggles with physical care or behavioral symptoms, for example, may have been replaced by struggles with guilt and loss. Former primary caregivers at home can benefit from a great deal of support by the rest of the family at this difficult time. It is also a good idea for the primary caregiver and other family members to continue to meet with the clinician, to help with the caregiver's adjustment to the placement.

CHAPTER 10

The End of the Journey:
New Beginnings

Gradually, but inexorably, the disease progresses. Eventually, the person with Alzheimer's moves into the final stages of the disease. Symptoms and signs of illness at this stage usually include the following:

- Recent memory is essentially absent.
- Language is largely incomprehensible or nonexistent.
- All instrumental activities of daily living have long since disappeared.
- No ability to perform any basic activities of daily living without assistance.
- Incontinence of bladder and usually of bowel.
- There are automatic actions, but little purposeful activity.
- Loss of recognition of familiar people, including close family members eventually.
- Very unsteady ambulation, or no longer able to ambulate at all.

At this point in the illness, it would seem reasonable that any treatments designed to keep the person alive longer should be discontinued.

- No transfer to the hospital for acute treatment (except to provide comfort, if this could not be done in the nursing home, or home setting).
- No antibiotics to be given for an infection (unless it is to provide comfort for a non-life-threatening condition).
- No tube feeding, once the person is no longer able or willing to take oral nourishment.
- Careful spoon feeding should be offered, but no forced feeding.
- Discontinue antidementia medications, one at a time, and observe for signs of worsening.

One of the most difficult symptoms at this stage is the loss of recognition of close family members. Even though there may be no intelligible language, the presence of a spouse or adult child may up to this point have led to a smile or other sign of pleasure. The afflicted person will look at a family member in a way that leads the family member to say, "She still knows who I am." It is impossible to tell if that is completely true, or if there is just enough of a sense of familiarity to produce the automatic reactions seen. Certainly, members of the Alzheimer's family have a strong need to believe that the individual continues to recognize them, and hold firmly to this view. Eventually, though, that sign of pleasure or sense of familiarity vanishes, and there remain no traces that the individual has any recognition whatsoever. When family members visit after this point, there is either no sign that the afflicted individual is aware of their presence, or that there is any difference between the family member and anyone else. Family members who have been in a state of anticipatory grief for some time now go into a new stage of mourning, feeling another deep sense of loss at no longer being recognized. There is no interaction of any kind, unless the person with Alzheimer's disease is physically stimulated in some way, and then he or she may react somewhat automatically. The final connections have all but dissolved.

Usually this loss of recognition does not come all at once; there is a progression through stages where there is no recognition one day, but there is recognition the next, or even at a different time on the same day. This variability can be confusing to the family member, but this is frequently how cognitive or functional abilities are lost: gradually and intermittently, until they are completely gone.

Many family members report that it is more difficult to visit the person in the nursing home when recognition has been lost. But most do continue to visit, out of habit, duty, a genuine desire to be close to their loved one, and perhaps a hope that today there will be a flicker of recognition. Others begin to visit less often at this point, for understandable reasons.

Such an afflicted person has entered end-stage dementia. Individuals with end-stage dementia are generally eligible for hospice care. Hospice can be extremely helpful with pain control and other late-stage physical symptoms. They also can provide a great deal of support for the family while the individual remains alive and for a period of time following death. The hospice nurse will generally visit the person at home or in the long-term care facility. For individuals enrolled in Medicare, the Medicare Hospice Benefit is substantial, and all care is provided at no additional cost to the patient or family. To have someone enrolled, the primary physician needs to ask hospice to consult, and if they agree with the appropriateness of the referral, this will happen. The overall goal of hospice is to provide "care, not cure"; while they offer extensive assistance with symptom control, there are no efforts to prolong life with intensive medical interventions. Prolonging the very late stages of this illness would seem to be of questionable value, since it is hard to imagine that the person with end-stage Alzheimer's disease continues to experience any positive quality of life.

DEATH

The most common cause of death in Alzheimer's disease is pneumonia. Persons with end-stage disease are often weak, emaciated, and lack the ability to successfully fight infections. They often lose the ability to swallow safely and can inhale food, or even saliva, into their windpipe, which settles in the lung and serves as a source of infection. End-stage patients are often poorly nourished due to poor food intake, and they may lack the ability to fight an infection. Of course, persons with late-stage Alzheimer's disease are usually quite elderly and may have a variety of other physical ailments that can be the cause of their demise. It is perhaps simply a matter of semantics whether people typically die *of* Alzheimer's or die *with* Alzheimer's. What is clear, however, is that Alzheimer's disease significantly increases the risk of other illnesses or injury that can be fatal in this population. This includes serious falls with head injury or fractured hip, infections, and other serious illnesses that can proceed undetected in those who are too demented to be able to report their symptoms.

AUTOPSY

Fewer autopsies are performed now than in the past, which is also true for autopsies of the brain of someone who has died with Alzheimer's disease. Many physicians will not request an autopsy from the surviving family of someone who has died with Alzheimer's disease, since the cause of death seems obvious and the physician understandably does not want to add any additional burdens to the grieving family. Even when an autopsy is requested, families often refuse, feeling that the procedure obviously will not benefit the deceased, and that a brain autopsy is needlessly mutilating. Yet the autopsy may offer considerable benefit to others, including the family.

While there is, as yet, no method of obtaining an exact diagnosis while someone is still living, looking at properly prepared slices of brain tissue under the microscope can determine whether the diagnosis is definitely Alzheimer's disease, as expected, or a different form of dementia. This may have genetic implications for the adult children of the deceased. We know, for example, that Alzheimer's disease occurs more frequently in offspring of persons with the disease, but that there are other forms of dementia that are not heritable. Experienced clinicians are accurate in their diagnostic assessment about 90% of the time; but one in 10 times, a different form of dementia is recognized from examining the brain tissue.

Another reason for an autopsy is that it can help bring some psychological closure to family members. Even when the autopsy confirms the diagnosis, family members will often feel that any uncertainties in their thinking (and nearly all experience uncertainty about the diagnosis, from time to time) will be clarified. Thus the autopsy may be a way to help family members move forward, after grieving their loss.

The other important reason autopsies can be valuable is to help future potential victims of the disease. When autopsies are performed by a "brain bank" (usually located at a university), tissue from the diseased brain can be studied by scientists who are working on a cure for the disease. It is always possible, therefore, that the small piece of tissue removed after autopsy and sent to a scientist studying Alzheimer's could be the key that unlocks the secret of the disease and leads to a cure or prevention. Some people with Alzheimer's are pleased to give consent to having a brain autopsy after their death, knowing that they are making an important contribution to medical science in general and to the cure of this disease in particular.

LIFE AFTER ALZHEIMER'S

The loss of the person with Alzheimer's disease is a long process. Frequently there have been years of anticipatory grief and a pervasive sense of ambiguous loss throughout the disease. Nevertheless, when death finally comes, there is usually a profound sadness that may even puzzle the Alzheimer's family caregiver, who thought all of the sadness must have already been experienced. There is also, much of the time, a sense of relief that the long struggle is finally over, for both the victim and the family. Many family members are reluctant to acknowledge this feeling, but the clinician should inquire about such emotions directly, after emphasizing that such a feeling is extremely common and understandable. Being able to verbalize openly about the relief experienced—both for the victim and for oneself—can be very helpful in moving normally through and beyond the grieving process.

For family members who were most involved in the daily care of the person with Alzheimer's, and who visited the nursing home regularly until the end, death creates a very real void. In Chapter 4, some of the differences between grief and depression were discussed. While family members are vulnerable to experiencing depression throughout the caregiving process, the risk of grief turning into a more painful and pathological state of depression at this time is very real. A family member whose grief has turned to depression may need to see a physician for antidepressant treatment.

Determining where grief ends and depression begins can be quite difficult. Some considerations for the clinician to keep in mind are as follows.

Grief

- Self-blame is minimal.
- Ability to experience pleasure remains, after the initial despair regarding the loss.
- Severity very gradually lessens over time, but can last months.
- Counseling or therapy can help; antidepressants generally do not help.

Depression

- Guilt over the death, or the relationship in general, is significant.
- Self-criticism (or blaming others) may be prominent.
- Ability to experience pleasure is lessened or absent even weeks or months after the loss.
- Tends to worsen over time; very rarely remits spontaneously.
- Counseling or therapy may help, but antidepressant medication is generally necessary to achieve remission.

DELAYED GRIEF

Some individuals feel only a sense of relief immediately following the death of a loved one with Alzheimer's disease. Their loved one may have had a particularly painful course of illness, emotionally, or may have suffered in other respects with concurrent physical ailments, for example. In these circumstances, that sense of relief is quite understandable. Nevertheless, it is always concerning when a member of the Alzheimer's family does not also feel some genuine sadness at the time of the death; this family member may be vulnerable to a serious delayed grief reaction at a later point. Delayed grief reactions can occur months or even years after the actual loss. People may avoid or delay their grief for a variety of reasons, but cannot escape it completely, even when there has been significant anticipatory grieving. Months following the death, the surviving loved one may have trouble moving on in terms of forming new relationships and getting involved in new activities to fill the time previously taken up by caregiving. A variety of physical symptoms may arise, which are concerning to the survivor but have no clear physical origin, including fatigue, various aches and pains, overeating, insomnia or excessive sleeping, and other ill-defined symptoms. Although such people deny feeling depressed, they do not really feel well either, but may not make any connection to the loss of their loved one with Alzheimer's disease. Later, a different loss—such as the death of a pet, a distant relative, or a public figure—may trigger a significant episode of depression. The sufferer may still not make a connection between these feelings and the death of the person with Alzheimer's—feeling only that the death was a relief after so much suffering—and it may be necessary for the clinician to guide the individual to make the connection between the current sadness and the loss of the parent or spouse with Alzheimer's. Frequently, it comes to the surface in conversation with the clinician that significant guilt is associated with the loss, although this is often heavily defended at least initially. Survivors feel they should have done more to help the person with the disease. Survivors may feel guilty about the nature of their relationship to the person with Alzheimer's before the disease, and even feel, on some level, that their feelings may have contributed to the disease in some way, even though they know objectively that this is not the case. Keeping these painful emotions below the surface may have been the unconscious motivation for avoiding the experience of grief at the time of the loss, but these feelings generally need to be explored and resolved with the clinician, so that these individuals can move forward with their lives.

It often seems that caregivers who have had healthy, mutually loving relationships with their now-deceased spouse or parent go through a very difficult grieving period, but gradually this resolves and the widow or adult child is able to return to living, sad about the loss, of course, but appreciative of the person who died and appreciative of the closeness they had. It is one of the ironies of grief that more ambivalent relationships—those in which there may have been significant closeness but a great deal of turmoil, as well—may be more difficult to grieve thoroughly and then move forward.

HELPING ONESELF BY HELPING OTHERS

One of the most valuable activities for the surviving caregiver is to share experiences with others who are at an earlier point of the same journey. Survivors who attended an Alzheimer's support group when their loved one was still living should be strongly encouraged to continue to attend, possibly after a brief hiatus, to deal with the acute stages of their loss. Those who never were able to find time to go to a support group should be encouraged to attend now. The survivor has an invaluable contribution to make, having been through the entire illness. Those who attend a support group after their loved one has died find the experience valuable. Other surviving family members find it useful to volunteer for an organization that assists families, such as the Alzheimer's Association, or to volunteer at a nursing home. There is no better training for working with Alzheimer's families than to have been through the entire process personally.

GETTING AWAY FROM ALZHEIMER'S DISEASE

It is also important to encourage surviving spouses and other members of the Alzheimer's family to become involved in activities that have nothing to do with Alzheimer's disease. Perhaps returning to an old hobby, given up because of the demands of the illness, or taking up a new one. Attending adult education classes or traveling with other seniors can be a valuable opportunity for the Alzheimer's widow or widower to reconnect to the community and to others at the same stage in life. Adult children of persons with the disease also need to resume their own lives, especially adult children who put their own young lives on hold to be available for the person with the disease.

FINDING MEANING

There is no doubt that the experience of being a caregiver takes a great deal from the Alzheimer's family caregiver. It takes, first and foremost, a loved one, slowly and painfully; it takes away time; it takes enormous sums of money; sometimes it takes away the caregiver's good health; and much else. In the end, it often seems that there is nothing left from which to go on and rebuild one's life. Yet it is critical for the Alzheimer's family caregiver to view the experience not simply as a saga of loss. It is essential for one's continued well-being from this point to find the positives in the experience. Caregivers certainly suffer during this long ordeal, but hopefully the experience also leads to significant growth. They have gained by giving as a caregivers. As noted earlier, people with Alzheimer's who are cared for by a loved one has given their loved one a gift, not just a burden. It is vitally important for Alzheimer's family caregivers to continue to recognize this and to value the gift they have received. Former caregivers need to find meaning in the experience and to discover how they have grown in the process. Many caregivers are surprised and pleased with the strength they discover in themselves. Others can claim to have learned patience and humility as a result of their role. Still others should take pride in having mastered the tasks that their afflicted loved one previously managed. And some Alzheimer's family caregivers have been able to forge an improved relationship with the person with the disease or with other family members because of the necessity of working together to care for the person with Alzheimer's.

All caregivers gain something in the process, although not all caregivers are able or willing to see how the experience has helped them, at least initially. Growth through adversity almost always takes place. As time goes on, and perhaps with the continuing help of the clinician, the caregiver and other members of the Alzheimer's family will be able to balance the losses and hardships they have experienced with pride and gratitude for the sense of personal growth that has come from this long and difficult journey.

APPENDIX: PHARMACOLOGIC TREATMENT OF THE COGNITIVE, FUNCTIONAL, AND BEHAVIORAL SYMPTOMS OF ALZHEIMER'S DISEASE

The treatment of Alzheimer's disease involves many interventions and interactions. Medication treatment is only one of these, and the medications currently available to treat the cognitive and functional symptoms of Alzheimer's disease are only modestly effective, at best. The more fundamental component of treatment always involves the low-tech, hands-on aspects of day-to-day care provided by the Alzheimer's family and other caregivers. While much of this book describes those interventions, this section focuses on medication treatment of the cognitive, functional, and behavioral symptoms of Alzheimer's disease. In general, optimal treatment involves a combination of antidementia medications, the occasional and judicious use of psychiatric medication for the various mood and behavioral symptoms that can develop, and the wide array of nonpharmacologic interventions and interactions described throughout this book.

TREATING THE COGNITIVE AND FUNCTIONAL SYMPTOMS OF ALZHEIMER'S DISEASE

The U.S. Food and Drug Administration (FDA) has determined that the following medications are safe and are effective in treating the cognitive and functional symptoms of Alzheimer's disease:

- **Donepezil.** Approved in 1997; a cholinesterase inhibitor. It is approved for mild, moderate, and severe Alzheimer's disease.
- **Rivastigmine.** Approved in 2000; a cholinesterase inhibitor. It is approved for mild to moderate Alzheimer's disease. It is also the only medication approved for dementia associated with Parkinson's disease. In 2007, rivastigmine became available in a transdermal (skin patch) form, in addition to oral preparations.
- **Galantamine.** Approved in 2001; a cholinesterase inhibitor. It is approved for mild to moderate Alzheimer's disease.
- **Memantine.** Approved in 2004; an NMDA inhibitor. It is approved for moderate to severe Alzheimer's disease.

Brand Name Versus Generic

When a so-called generic version of a medication is available, this means that the patent on the original compound has expired and other companies in addition to the original manufacturer are permitted to produce the drug, selling it by the generic name. This generally means that the medication is available at a significantly lower cost. In most states, pharmacies are required to dispense a generic instead of the more expensive brand name alternative, unless the physician specifically requests the brand name version. Most insurance companies will also require that generics be given when available.

As of this writing, donepezil, galantamine and rivastigmine are available generically.. Memantine can only be obtained as the brand Namenda.

Cholinesterase Inhibitors

Donepezil, rivastigmine, and galantamine are cholinesterase inhibitors. These medications exert their effect, at least in part, by inhibiting (blocking) the action of the enzyme acetylcholinesterase, which breaks down the protein acetylcholine. Acetylcholine is a neurotransmitter (chemical messenger) that operates at the synapse (junction) of one nerve cell with the next, permitting the transmission of a nerve impulse from the presynaptic neuron to the postsynaptic neuron, and thus through the brain. There are many neurotransmitters in the brain, but acetylcholine is a critical one in areas concerned with learning and memory. In Alzheimer's disease and some other dementias, the amount of this neurotransmitter available decreases significantly, and therefore these learning and memory circuits are unable to function normally. Acetylcholine itself cannot be ingested, as it would be inactivated or destroyed before it reached the nervous system. Therefore, the only way to increase acetylcholine levels is to interfere with its normal metabolic breakdown (by blocking acetylcholinesterase).

While a greatly diminished supply of acetylcholine is a cardinal feature of Alzheimer's disease, it is only one of aspect of the disease's very complex pathology. For this reason, raising acetylcholine by giving cholinesterase inhibitors is often helpful but is certainly not a cure.

Overall, each of the cholinesterase inhibitors is about equally effective. However, some individuals may respond better to one than another, for unexplained reasons. There is no firm evidence that changing from one cholinesterase inhibitor to another, if the first seems to no longer be effective, will produce benefit, but it may be something to consider.

Side Effects of Cholinesterase Inhibitors

Overall, cholinesterase inhibitors are safe and reasonably well tolerated when taken according to the guidelines given below. The most common side effects of cholinesterase inhibitors are gastrointestinal: nausea, diarrhea, stomach distress, loss of appetite, weight loss, queasiness, a feeling of bloating or gas, or vomiting. These side effects can be lessened or avoided by giving low doses initially and taking the medication on a full stomach, with or following a meal. A small percentage of individuals are unable to tolerate the gastrointestinal side effects of the medication.

Other less common side effects are leg cramps, which come irregularly, often when the patient is in bed. Other side effects include vivid dreams or even nightmares. Nightmares can be frequent and disturbing enough to consider terminating the medication, but this is rare.

An important adverse effect of cholinesterase inhibitors is bradycardia (abnormally slow heart rate), which can cause dizziness, fainting, falling, and potential injury. Cholinesterase inhibitors should be avoided if there is a cardiac conduction disturbance or a very slow heart rate. Other possible side effects include insomnia, dizziness, exacerbation of asthma or chronic obstructive pulmonary disease, and rhinorrhea (runny nose).

If a dose is missed, it should be skipped. If the medication is stopped for any reason for more than a week, it may be necessary to resume at a lower dose, initially.

Rivastigmine Patch

One of the cholinesterase inhibitors, rivastigmine, is now available in a transdermal (skin patch) form. This patch is applied to the chest, upper arm, or back once a day. There is a significantly lower level of gastrointestinal side effects with rivastigmine patch compared to the oral agents, and it may be a good choice for someone who is unable to tolerate an oral medication because of those side effects. It may be preferred by a person who dislikes taking pills or is unable to do so. Skin rash can develop but is not common.

No more than one cholinesterase inhibitor should be given at a time, as this can lead to toxic reactions.

N-Methyl-D-Aspartate Receptor Antagonists

Memantine is the only *N*-methyl-D-aspartate (NMDA) receptor antagonist currently available for the treatment of Alzheimer's disease. Memantine works by a complex mechanism of action that reduces glutamatergic excitotoxicity in the neuron. This mode of action is completely different from that of the cholinesterase inhibitors, which is why it is possible (and often desirable) to use both memantine and a cholinesterase inhibitor at the same time.

While cholinesterase inhibitors exert their effect on neurons that utilize the neurotransmitter acetylcholine, memantine acts on a different neurotransmitter, glutamate. The glutamate system is prominent in the learning and memory areas of the brain. Memantine lessens the effect of excess glutamate (which occurs when there are damaged brain cells) at synapses that utilize the NMDA receptor. This facilitates more effective transmission of neural impulses. Memantine may also help preserve the life of neurons, by limiting the excessive flow of calcium into nerve cells.

Memantine has been approved by the FDA for moderate to severe Alzheimer's disease.

Memantine Side Effects

Memantine has relatively few side effectss. It can be mildly constipating; this effect can offset the gastrointestinal hyperactivity caused by cholinesterase inhibitors, lessening the incidence of diarrhea or other gastrointestinal side effects caused by a cholinesterase inhibitor. Other adverse effects include headache, dizziness, somnolence, and, occasionally, worsened confusion or agitation. These last effects are usually quite short lived but can certainly be unsettling for the caregiver. Temporarily lowering the dose will frequently improve the situation, but not always.

Memantine is not significantly metabolized by the liver, like most medications, but is excreted essentially unchanged by the kidneys. Therefore, individuals with significant impairment of kidney function may need to take a lower dose. Persons with renal failure (not on dialysis) should not use memantine at all.

There are few drug interactions, but other medications that also act on NMDA receptors should not be taken at the same time, including amantadine (Symmetrel); rimantadine (Flumadine), ketamine, and methadone. Other opiates are permissible. Over-the-counter cough preparations that contain dextromethorphan should be avoided as dextromethorphan is also an NMDA inhibitor.

Starting and Maintaining Memantine

The manufacturer and the FDA recommend a gradual titration when initiating the medication: 5 mg per day the first week; 5 mg twice a day the second week; 10 mg in the morning and 5 mg in the evening for the third week; and then 10 mg twice a day, which is the usual maintenance dose.

WHAT TO EXPECT FROM ANTIDEMENTIA MEDICATIONS

Slowing the Decline

There is no cure for Alzheimer's disease, or for most other types of dementia. Most forms of dementia, in particular Alzheimer's disease, are progressive: from the time they begin until the time of death, they relentlessly worsen. In general, the overall effect of antidementia medications is to slow the progress of the disease.

Degree of Effectiveness

Overall, the effect of these medications is relatively modest. Some individuals have a very positive response, with improvement in symptoms for some time; others have a noticeable but not dramatic response; some appear to have little if any benefit; and some individuals have no discernible response to the drugs, at all. There is absolutely no way to tell, ahead of time, who will respond to the medications and who will not.

Effect on Survival

There is no definitive evidence that antidementia medications keep people alive longer. Rather, it seems that they may help keep people cognitively well longer, more functional longer, and with a better overall quality of life.

Duration of Benefit

Antidementia medications tend to have a peak effect in 2–3 months after reaching a therapeutic dose. The myth that the medications cease to work after a year and should be stopped at that point is entirely false. This impression is based on the fact that the early studies of cholinesterase inhibitors demonstrated a gain in cognitive ability initially, with a gradual decline thereafter, with the patient returning to baseline in about 1 year. Subjects who were given an inactive placebo were significantly worse at the end of that year, however, making it clear that being no better, but no worse, after 1 year is actually an important therapeutic effect in a progressive illness such as Alzheimer's.

Studies (Rountree et al., 2009; Atri et al., 2008) have suggested that antidementia medications exert their effect for at least several years, although exactly how long they should be given has not been determined by systematic research.

How to Determine if the Medication Is Working

Sometimes, it is obvious; individuals are sharper, more attentive, and more interactive. They remember better, are able to perform tasks they could not perform before, and overall seem to have more initiative. While one always hopes for such a positive effect, this occurs less than half the time, unfortunately. More frequently, some slight gains may be noted initially, which seem to fade; or there is no discernible benefit. In this situation, the medication may be slowing down the progression of the disease or may be having little or no effect at all. Unfortunately there is no way to be sure about this over any short period of time. Ideally a person with Alzheimer's disease should take antidementia medications for a minimum of 6 months to 1 year to adequately assess the overall effectiveness of the treatment. At the end of this time, if the medication is having the desired effect, there should be little or no overall decline in the person's condition. In untreated cases of Alzheimer's disease, individuals are noticeably worse after 6 months to a year. If someone has been taking both a cholinesterase inhibitor and memantine, the improvement is likely due to the combination, and it may be impossible to sort out which has been more helpful. Determining whether or not the medication has been helping can be difficult and should be done in consultation with the prescribing physician.

Combination Therapy

A number of studies (e.g., Lopez et al., 2009; Atri et al., 2008; Tariot et al., 2004) suggest that the combination of a cholineste-

rase inhibitor (donepezil, galantamine, or rivastigmine) plus memantine is generally the most effective regimen in slowing the
decline of cognition and function.

Are Antidementia Drugs Worthwhile?

The limited effects of antidementia medications have led to debate as to whether or not the drugs are worthwhile. However,
since it is not possible to know in advance if a particular individual
will have a robust response to antidementia medication, an average (modest) response, or no discernible response, it would seem
that antidementia medications should at least be given an adequate therapeutic trial, if the cost can be managed, and there are
no or minimal side effects. Most patients and families feel that any
intervention that may slow down this devastating disease process
is certainly worth trying, at least.

Discontinuing Antidementia Medications

Some physicians will continue antidementia medications indefinitely, while others will take a more active role in trying to assess
their continued value. The clinician can be helpful to the family in
determining whether the antidementia medications have continuing value and can suggest that a discussion with the physician
about their continued role is in order. While there are no firm
guidelines in the medical literature as to when antidementia medications should be discontinued, once the individual reaches the
very late stages of dementia, it may be reasonable to discontinue
these medications. If a decision is made to discontinue antidementia medications at any point, it should be done in consultation with
the prescriber. If the person with Alzheimer's is on two different
antidementia medications, only one medication should be stopped
at a time, watching for any unexpected or untoward effects. Obvious clinical worsening can occur within 2 weeks of stopping an
antidementia medication, even when all were convinced that the
drug was no longer having any meaningful effect. If there is a loss
of cognitive or functional abilities after discontinuing a medication, this decline can usually be stabilized by restarting the medi-

cation rapidly. However, the abilities that have been lost may or may not be regained.

INTERVENTIONS OF UNCERTAIN VALUE

There was hope that large doses of the omega-3 fatty acid DHA, which is found in cold-water fish and other foods, might slow the progression of Alzheimer's disease, but unfortunately a large, multisite study of DHA(Quinn JF, 2010) is has shown that the substance is of little or no value in persons who already have the disease. It may be somewhat helpful for those with very mild degrees of cognitive decline.

Various B vitamins have been touted as helpful in preventing or slowing cognitive decline (Smith, 2008) while others have not found this to be true (Ford et al., 2010) Others feel that exogenous antioxidant vitamins, such as vitamin C and vitamin E, may be helpful (Devore et al., 2010), but the evidence for this is inconclusive, and other studies (Miller et al., 2005) have shown that high doses of vitamin E may be associated with an increased risk of death.

Some studies have found that cholesterol-lowering medications (statins) may lower the risk of developing Alzheimer's (Wolozin et al., 2000), but other studies have not found this to be true (McGuinness et al., 2009). Of course, these agents may be very useful in reducing the risk of cardiovascular disease in those who have elevated cholesterol.

In the past, estrogen was recommended for both preventing and treating Alzheimer's, but any benefit is outweighed by the risks now recognized to be associated with this hormone treatment, and estrogen is no longer recommended for Alzheimer's disease. Similarly, it was hoped that nonsteroidal anti-inflammatory medications (NSAIDs) such as ibuprofen might lower the risk of developing Alzheimer's (Veld, 2001). More recent studies have not found this to be true, and heavy use of NSAIDs may increase, not decrease, the risk of developing Alzheimer's disease (Sonnen, 2010).

A variety of other agents, such as curcumin, phosphatidylser-ine, coenzyme Q10, huperzine A, and medium-chain triglyceride oil have been promoted, but no firm scientific evidence exists that these are helpful. Acupuncture has also been promoted as a treatment for Alzheimer's, but again there is no definite scientific evidence that it is helpful for this condition.

A recent, definitive clinical trial involving ginkgo biloba, which had been touted for many years as a useful treatment for Alzheimer's disease, has found that ginkgo offers no benefit for Alzheimer's disease, unfortunately (Snitz et al., 2009).

Clearly, the inconsistency of the evidence for these interventions makes it clear that much remains to be learned about what will help delay or prevent Alzheimer's disease.

CLINICAL TRIALS

Many new medications are in various stages of research and development, although there have been a number of recent late-stage failures. Clinical trials are research studies in which new medications that have already been proven to be safe are tested for effectiveness. Up-to-date information about current clinical trials in Alzheimer's disease and related disorders can be obtained by visiting the NIH Clinical Trials Web site, http://clinicaltrials.gov/.

ANTIDEMENTIA MEDICATIONS FOR OTHER DEMENTIAS

Vascular Dementia

There is limited information in the literature about the effectiveness of antidementia medications for the treatment of vascular dementia. However, as noted above, it is often impossible to determine whether Alzheimer's disease pathology is also present. The majority of demented persons with vascular disease of the brain also have the characteristic plaques and tangles of Alzheimer's disease. Therefore, it would be appropriate to treat these individuals with medications that have been shown to be effective with

Alzheimer's disease—cholinesterase inhibitors and memantine—and indeed, clinical experience suggests that these are often helpful.

Lewy Body Dementia

Persons with Lewy body dementia do appear to respond to anti-dementia medications, although such medications do not help the physical (parkinsonian) symptoms of the disease. Antiparkinson medications such as levodopa/carbidopa are variably helpful for the motor symptoms of Lewy body dementia but do not help the cognitive symptoms.

Parkinson's Dementia

Only one medication is currently approved by the FDA for the treatment of dementia associated with Parkinson's disease—rivastigmine. While it can be quite helpful in lessening or temporarily stabilizing the cognitive symptoms, it certainly does not cure them, and the disease will continue to progress, unfortunately. Medications used to treat the motor symptoms of Parkinson's disease—for example, levodopa/carbidopa, benztropine, and the like—do not help cognition and will, in fact, often worsen the cognitive symptoms of the disease, so careful clinical management is needed.

Frontotemporal Dementia

Unfortunately, medications that have been shown to be effective for Alzheimer's disease have not been found to be effective for frontotemporal dementia. Because behavioral symptoms are prominent, many individuals with this dementia are treated with psychiatric medications, and while they may be helpful in bringing some of the more troublesome symptoms under control, they do not help to slow down the progression of the disease.

MANAGING MOOD AND BEHAVIORAL ISSUES

Nonmedication Interventions for Mood and Behavioral Problems

It is always best to try nonpharmacologic approaches to improving behavioral problems, before resorting to drugs, although sometimes medications may be needed, along with other techniques, to deal with a behavioral symptom. It is not a failure on the part of the individual or the family if psychiatric medications become necessary; it merely reflects how difficult and distressing these problems can be, and it is a sign of wisdom and good judgment to be willing to use any tool necessary to try to improve a difficult situation.

Some individuals or families—and indeed some therapists and even some nonpsychiatric medical practitioners—have strong prejudices against the use of psychotropic medications in general, or for people with Alzheimer's disease in particular. This is frequently based on having known someone who responded poorly to psychotropics, or someone who was overmedicated and suffered adverse effects or a loss of functional abilities as a result. Such situations are most unfortunate, indeed, but such mishaps are definitely not the inevitable result of using psychotropic medications. Others may feel that doctors who prescribe psychotropic medications for people with Alzheimer's necessarily devalue the importance of nonpharmacologic interventions for mood and behavior. While that may apply to certain medical practitioners, it is certainly not true for all. Indeed, the best approach for managing difficult mood and behavioral symptoms is often a combination of careful environmental intervention along with judicious use of medication.

Considering Medications for Mood and Behavioral Symptoms of Alzheimer's Disease

Even though it may generally be best to try to avoid medications for mood and behavioral symptoms, they may be helpful at times. The person with Alzheimer's disease and the family members should feel no sense of shame about this, or feel that if they only tried harder, the medications would not be necessary. One would certainly not feel that way about taking medication for hypertension, kidney disease, or osteoporosis. Mood and behavioral symptoms in dementia are extraordinarily common, painful complications of the disease. Psychotropic medications can be helpful at times, improving quality of life for both the patient and caregiver.

Some general considerations:

- If there is a change in behavior, or the individual appears particularly distressed and cannot express what the problem is, it may be important to rule out any acute medical problems such as a urinary tract or respiratory infection, or pain. Undiagnosed and untreated pain is common in persons with dementia who are no longer able to communicate their needs verbally.
- It is necessary to assess the nature and severity of the symptoms, to determine if nonpharmacologic approaches would be helpful, whether or not medications are also used.
- In making a decision about the use of psychotropic medications, one should consider the risks of the medications, the likelihood that they will be helpful, the severity of the symptoms, and the risks (e.g., in terms of suffering, possibility of harm) of not using medication to treat the symptoms.
- All psychiatric medications have potential side effects, including the possibility of worsening cognition and functional abilities during the time they are used. However, many mood or behavioral symptoms themselves can cause impairment in cognition and functioning, which could be improved by adequate treatment.
- The lowest possible dose of medication should be used, but it is important to ensure that the amount given is an effective dose. Very often, persons with dementia are treated with subtherapeutic doses of psychotropic medications for fear that higher doses will cause complications. Giving an ineffectively low dose of a medication is worse than not using the medication at all.
- Once someone has been started on a psychotropic medication, there should be regular evaluations to determine how long the medication will be needed and if the dosage is optimal. Dosing needs can change (up or down) over the course of time. Some medications should be used for lengthy periods; others should be used only when the symptoms are acute. The decision about stopping a psychotropic medication should always involve the physician who prescribed the medication.

• All antipsychotic medications, such as quetiapine (Seroquel), olanzapine (Zyprexa), risperidone (Risperdal), haloperidol (Haldol), and others are required by the FDA to carry a black box warning about their use in older individuals with dementia, because numerous studies have shown that the use of antipsychotic medications in persons with dementia is associated with a small but statistically significant increase in sudden death, usually from cardiovascular or other causes. In addition, other significant adverse reactions can occur with this class of medications. While they should be avoided if at all possible in people with Alzheimer's disease, occasionally, when all else has failed and the person is in considerable distress or is a danger to himself or others, a physician may feel it is necessary to prescribe an antipsychotic agent. If so, this should be done cautiously, at the lowest effective dose, and the patient should be monitored closely while being treated with the medication.

MEDICATION FOR SPECIFIC BEHAVIORAL ISSUES

Aggressiveness

It is sometimes possible to utilize medications to help reduce aggressiveness, along with appropriate behavioral and environmental approaches. The use of medications for aggression should depend on a thorough evaluation by a physician or other medical practitioner experienced in this area. Medications that are sometimes useful for aggressiveness include the following.

Serotonin Reuptake Inhibitors

Serotonin reuptake inhibitors (SSRIs), primarily used for depression and anxiety, can also be substantially helpful with mild to moderate irritability. SSRIs include:

• Sertraline
• Citalopram
• Escitalopram

Paroxetine, a widely used SSRI, should be avoided in people with Alzheimer's disease, because it has anticholinergic properties. People with Alzheimer's already have a significant diminution of achetylcholine, and anticholinergic agents can potentially worsen memory or cause delirium. In addition, paroxetine has many interactions with other medications, causing unpredictable elevations in blood levels.

Fluoxetine should also be avoided, if possible. While not anticholinergic, it also interacts with many other medications and has a very long half-life so that discontinuing the medication and waiting for it to be fully out of the system can take a number of weeks.

Trazodone

Although trazodone was originally introduced as an antidepressant and is still occasionally used to elevate mood, it requires relatively large doses that are not easily tolerated by older individuals. However, trazodone also has a significant calming or sedating effect and can be very helpful in treating agitation or anxiety, either as a routine medication given several times a day or as an as-needed (prn) medication when anxiety or agitation develops infrequently or unexpectedly. Trazodone is also a very safe and effective medication to assist with sleep. It is not habit forming, unlike most other sleep agents.

Buspirone

Buspirone is a nonbenzodiazepine antianxiety medication. It is also useful in some cases of agitation or aggressiveness in persons with dementia. While it is only variably helpful, it is usually worth considering because it is safe and has few side effects.

Mood Stabilizers

Medications in the category of mood stabilizers include the following:

- Valproic acid
- Carbamazepine
- Lamotrigine

These medications are primarily anticonvulsants but have been shown to be helpful as mood stabilizers for bipolar patients. They are often helpful in lessening agitation or aggression in persons with dementia.

Benzodiazepines and Antipsychotics

Benzodiazepines (lorazepam and the like) should be used sparingly, if at all. Likewise, antipsychotic agents such as haloperidol or quetiapine should be avoided for the treatment of agitation except under very extreme and unusual circumstances, since these medications have been associated with an increased risk of sudden death from cardiovascular and other complications in older persons with dementia. When all else has failed, the person with Alzheimer's is in distress from the symptoms, there is danger to the person with dementia or others because of the behavior, and if the family gives informed, written consent, it may be appropriate to cautiously utilize antipsychotic medications, in the lowest possible doses for the shortest period of time, and with careful documentation. Occasionally, a physician will give antipsychotic medications when other interventions may be more appropriate or effective. Under these circumstances, the clinician may want to suggest that the caregiver discuss this with the treating physician and request that an alternate medication be used if at all possible.

It can be difficult if not impossible to know what medication will be most effective for a given episode of aggressiveness. The physician may make a choice based on some characteristics of the symptoms, but treating agitation with medication is largely trial and error. If one particular medication is not effective, in adequate doses given for adequate amounts of time, it may be appropriate to gradually discontinue that medication and try a different one. As always, it is very important to make only one change in the medication regimen at a time; otherwise, it becomes impossible to know which change is helping (if the symptoms are improving) or making the situation worse (if there are side effects).

Anxiety

If anxiety is intense or unremitting it may be appropriate to consider medication. The most effective and safe medications to use for anxiety include the following:

- SSRIs such as sertraline, citalopram, or escitalopram.
- Serotonin-norepinephrine reuptake inhibitors (SNRIs), such as venlafaxine, that have been approved by the FDA for the treatment of anxiety as well as of depression may be helpful, although they are usually not the first group of medications considered for anxiety in dementia.
- Buspirone can be useful in calming anxiety, because it is not habit forming and individuals do not develop tolerance for it. Unfortunately, it is not always effective, but it is worth considering.
- Trazodone: While SSRIs, SNRIs, and buspirone need to be given regularly, every day, to be effective, trazodone can be given as prn only, when anxiety appears to be increasing, or it can be scheduled at times of the day when anxiety is a common problem, such as late afternoon.

Benzodiazepines such as lorazepam should be used very sparingly, if at all, due to the risk of adverse effects. Antipsychotic agents should not be given simply for anxiety, because of the risks associated with these medications.

Apathy

A variety of medications are sometimes used to attempt to treat apathy, with variable success. They include the following:

- Bupropion, a stimulating antidepressant.
- Methylphenidate and other stimulants.
- Antidementia medications (cholinesterase inhibitors or memantine), which are given for their primary effects on cognition and function, but may help diminish apathy in some people with Alzheimer's disease.

As is often the case, behavioral interventions may be more beneficial than medications in dealing with apathy.

Depression

Antidepressants can be an extremely valuable intervention for the person with Alzheimer's disease, although not every expression of sadness should be seen as a call for medication.

There is a variety of antidepressants; overall, there is no consensus that one is more effective than another, and different individuals may respond well to one and poorly to another, for unclear reasons. If someone does not respond well to one, a different one should be tried.

The most commonly used antidepressants used in people with Alzheimer's disease are the following:

- SSRIs such as sertraline, citalopram, and escitalopram
- SNRIs, including venlafaxine and duloxetine
- Mirtazapine
- Bupropion

Disinhibited Behaviors

Most disinhibited behaviors do not respond to medication. However, males who are sexually disinhibited and aggressive may respond to paroxetine, an SSRI that can cause a significant loss of libido. Other SSRIs may have similar effects, but paroxetine may have the greatest impact on sexual drive. Other men with sexual aggressiveness are sometimes treated with estrogen or other antiandrogenic hormones to decrease libido. There are only anecdotal reports that these interventions are sometimes effective; there have been no randomized controlled trials. However, given the significant negative effect these behaviors can have and their poor response to other, nonpharmacologic interventions, a trial of medication may be warranted.

Hallucinations

If hallucinations are extremely disturbing to the person with Alzheimer's disease or lead to dangerous behaviors (such as running into traffic to try to meet a hallucinated person), the use of medications may be warranted. Unfortunately, there are no medications that are particularly helpful with hallucinations other than antipsychotic medications. As noted, these need to be used only when absolutely necessary, and then with caution because of the increased risk of sudden death. In addition, it is important that the prescribing physician have a careful discussion about these medications with the family of the hallucinating person to review the risks and benefits of their use, or nonuse, and to obtain informed consent from the person with health care power of attorney, as well as from the individual who is hallucinating, if that is possible.

Antipsychotic medications used for hallucinations include the following:

- Haloperidol
- Quetiapine
- Risperidone
- Olanzapine
- Aripiprazole

It is important that there be periodic attempts to discontinue the medication when the symptoms no longer seem to be a problem.

Sleep

Medications for sleep may or may not be useful and should only be used if the sleep disturbance is distressing to the patient or if the caregiver is unable to sleep because of wandering or other behaviors at night. Then, only safe medications, such as melatonin or trazodone, should be used if at all possible. Only if absolutely necessary should the person with Alzheimer's be given any of the medications that are marketed for sleep, such as zolpidem, as these may be habit forming and may worsen cognition or lead to gait unsteadiness. Benzodiazepines such as lorazepam are sometimes given for sleep, but because lorazepam is short acting, the individual may not be able to remain asleep throughout the night. Longer-acting benzodiazepines such as clonazepam should be avoided in the elderly because they can accumulate and cause adverse effects. It is also important to avoid over-the-counter medications for sleep. Such aids generally contain diphenhydramine or another anticholinergic drug, which can cause significant confusion or paradoxical agitation or delirium in persons with Alzheimer's disease.

One of the greatest problems with sleep medication is that the individual (and perhaps the family member administering it) becomes psychologically, if not physiologically, dependent on the medication very quickly, and it becomes very difficult to discontinue the medication. It is not clear if the actual drug is needed to sleep, or merely the idea of taking the drug. Sometimes, replacing a sleep aid with plain acetaminophen can be useful, and many older people feel that one or two Tylenol at bedtime do help them sleep.

Sundowning

If sundowning is a daily event and occurs at a predictable time, it can be quite useful to give a low dose of trazodone every day, before the symptoms begin. Otherwise, an as-needed dose of medication can be given if and when the behaviors start. If the medication is given immediately when the symptoms start (or right before), it is more likely to be helpful. If one waits until the individual is very agitated or confused, the medication may be too little, too late, and have a negligible effect. Medications other than trazodone are occasionally used, but trazodone is the most reliably helpful for this problem, has few side effects when given in appropriate doses, and is inexpensive.

READINGS & RESOURCES

REFERENCES

2011 Alzheimer's Disease Facts and Figures. Chicago: Alzheimer's Association, 2011.

American Psychiatric Association. (1994). *Diagnostic and statistical manual of mental disorders* (4th ed.). Washington, DC: American Psychiatric Association.

Atri, A., Shaughnessy, L. W., Locascio, J. J., & Growdon, J. H. (2008). Long-term course and effectiveness of combination therapy in Alzheimer disease *Alzheimer Disease and Associated Disorders*, 22(3), 209–21.

Beeri, M, S., Schmeidler, J., Lesser, G. T., Maroukian, M., West, R., Leung, S., Wysocki, M., Perl, D.P., Purohit, D.P., & Haroutunian, V. (2011, March 31). Corticosteroids, but not NSAIDs, are associated with less Alzheimer neuropathology. *Neurobiology of Aging*, epub ahead of print.

Boss, P. (1999). *Ambiguous Loss: Learning to live with unresolved grief*. Cambridge, MA: Harvard University Press.

Ceravolo R., Rossi, C., Kiferle, L., & Bonuccelli, U. (2010). Nonmotor symptoms in Parkinson's disease: The dark side of the moon. *Future Neurology*, 5(6): 851–71.

Chaudhuri, K. R., Healy, D. G., & Schapira, A. H. (2006). Nonmotor symptoms of Parkinson's disease: Diagnosis and management *Lancet Neurology*, 5(3), 235–45.

Devore, E. E., Grodstein, F., van Rooij, F. J., Hofman, A., Stampfer, M. J., Witteman, J. C., & Breteler, M. M. (2010). Dietary antioxidants and long-term risk of dementia. *Archives of Neurology*, 67(7), 819–25.

Ford, A. H., Flicker, L., Alfonso, H., Thomas, J., Clarnette, R., Martins, R., & Almeida, O. P. (2010). Vitamins B(12), B(6), and folic acid for cognition in older men. *Neurology*, 75(17), 1540–47.

in t' Veld, B.A., Ruitenberg, A., Hofman, A., Launer, L. J., van Duijn, C. M., Stijnen, T., Breteler, M. M., & Stricker, B. H. (2001). Nonsteroidal antiinflammatory drugs and the risk of Alzheimer's disease. *New England Journal of Medicine*, 345(21), 1515–21.

Kosunen, O., Soininen, H., Paljärvi, L., Heinonen, O., Talasniemi, S., & Riekkinen, P. J. Sr. (1996). Diagnostic accuracy of Alzheimer's disease: a neuropathological study. *Acta Neuropathologica*, 91(2), 185–93.

Lopez, O. L., Becker, J. T., Wahed, A. S., Saxton, J., Sweet, R. A., Wolk, D. A., Klunk, W., & Dekosky, S. T. (2009). Long-term effects of the concomitant use of memantine with cholinesterase inhibition in Alzheimer disease. *Journal of Neurology, Neurosurgery and Psychiatry*, 80(6), 600–7.

Mace, N. L., & Rabins, P. V. (2006). *The 36-hour day: A family guide to caring for persons with Alzheimer's disease, related dementing illnesses, and memory loss in later life* (4th ed.). Baltimore: Johns Hopkins University Press.

Marin, D. B., Green, C. R., Schmeidler, J., Harvey, P. D., Lawlor, B. A., Ryan, T. M., Aryan, M., Davis, K. L., & Mohs, R. C. (1997). Noncognitive disturbances in Alzheimer's disease: frequency, longitudinal course, and relationship to cognitive symptoms. *Journal of the American Geriatrics Society,* 45(11), 1331–8.

McGuinness, B., Craig, D., Bullock, R., & Passmore, P. (2009). Statins for the prevention of dementia. *Cochrane Database of Systematic Reviews,* Issue 2.

Miller, E. R., Pastor-Barriuso, R., Dalal, D., Riemersma, R. A., Appel, L. J., & Guallar, E, (2005). Meta-analysis: High-dosage vitamin E supplementation may increase all-cause mortality. *Annals of Internal Medicine,* 142(1), 37–46

Querfurth, H. W., & LaFerla, F. M. (2010). Alzheimer's disease. *New England Journal of Medicine,* 362, 329–44.

Quinn, J. F., Raman, R., Thomas, R. G., Yurko-Mauro, K., Nelson, E. B., Van Dyck, C., Galvin, J. E., Emond, J., Jack, C. R., Jr., Weiner, M., Shinto, L., & Aisen, P. S. (2010). Docosahexaenoic acid supplementation and cognitive decline in Alzheimer disease: a randomized trial. *Journal of the American Medical Association,* 304(17), 1903–11.

Rountree, S. D., Chan, W., Pavlik, V. N., Darby, E. J., Siddiqui, S., & Doody, R. S. (2009). Persistent treatment with cholinesterase inhibitors and/or memantine slows clinical progression of Alzheimer disease. *Alzheimer's Research and Therapy,* 21(2), 7.

Smith, A. D. (2008). The worldwide challenge of the dementias: a role for B vitamins and homocysteine? *Food and Nutrition Bulletin,* 29(2 Suppl), 143–72.

Snitz, B. E., O'Meara, E. S., Carlson, M. C., Arnold, A. M., Ives, D. G., Rapp, S. R., Saxton, J., Lopez, O. L., Dunn, L. O., Sink, K. M., & DeKosky, S. T. (2009). Ginkgo Evaluation of Memory (GEM) study investigators. Ginkgo biloba for preventing cognitive decline in older adults: a randomized trial. *Journal of the American Medical Association,* 302(24), 2663–70.

Sonnen, J. A., Larson, E. B., Walker, R. L., Haneuse, S., Crane, P. K., Gray, S. L., Breitner, J. C., & Montine, T. J. (2010). Nonsteroidal anti-inflammatory drugs are associated with increased neuritic plaques. *Neurology.* 75(13), 1203–10.

Tariot, P. N., Farlow, M. R., Grossberg, G. T., Graham, S. M., McDonald, S., & Gergel, I. (2004). Memantine study group. Memantine treatment in patients with moderate to severe Alzheimer disease. *Journal of the American Medical Association,* 291(3), 317–24.

The Shriver report: A woman's nation takes on Alzheimer's. (2010). New York: Free Press.

Wolozin, B., Kellman, K.., Rousseau, R.., Celesia, G. G., & Siegel, G. (2000). Decreased prevalence of Alzheimer disease associated with 3-Hydroxy-3-Methyglutaryl Coenzyme A reductase inhibitors. *Archives of Neurology,* 57, 1439–43.

SELECTED READINGS FOR CLINICIANS

Agüera-Ortiz, L., Frank-Garcia, A., Gil, P., et al. (2010). Clinical progression of moderate-to-severe Alzheimer's disease and caregiver burden: A 12-month multicenter prospective observational study. *International Psychogeriatrics,* 22(8), 1265–1279.

Boss, P. (1999). *Ambiguous loss: Learning to live with unresolved grief.* Cambridge, MA: Harvard University Press.

Dias, A., Dewey, M. E., D'Souza, J., et al. (2008). The effectiveness of a home care program for supporting caregivers of persons with dementia in developing countries: A randomised controlled trial from Goa, India. *PLoS ONE, 3*(6), e2333. doi:10.1371/journal.pone.0002333.

Frank, J. B. (2008). Evidence for grief as the major barrier faced by Alzheimer's caregivers: A qualitative analysis. *American Journal of Alzheimer's Disease and Other Dementias, 22*(6), 516–527.

Gaugler, J. E., Roth, D. L., Haley, W. E., & Mittelman, M. S. (2008). Can counseling and support reduce burden and depressive symptoms in caregivers of people with Alzheimer's disease during the transition to institutionalization? Results from the New York University caregiver intervention study. *Journal of the American Geriatrics Society, 56*(3), 421–428.

Gautier, S. (Ed.). (2006). *Clinical diagnosis and management of Alzheimer's disease* (3rd ed.). London: Informa Healthcare.

Meuser, T. M., & Marwit, S. J. (2001). A comprehensive, stage-sensitive model of grief in dementia caregiving. *Gerontologist, 41*(5), 658–670

Mittelman, M. S., Epstein, C., & Pierzchala, A. (2003). *Counseling the Alzheimer's caregiver: A resource for health care professionals.* Chicago: American Medical Association.

Mittelman, M. S., Haley, W. E., Clay, O. J., & Roth, D. L. (2006). Improving caregiver well-being delays nursing home placement of patients with Alzheimer disease. *Neurology, 67,* 1592–1599.

Mittelman, M. S., Roth, D. L., Clay, O. J., & Haley, W. E. (2007). Preserving health of Alzheimer caregivers: Impact of a spouse caregiver intervention. *American Journal of Geriatric Psychiatry, 15*(9), 780–789.

Nichols, L. O., Chang, C., Lummus, A., et al. 2008. The cost-effectiveness of a behavior intervention with caregivers of patients with Alzheimer's disease. *Journal of the American Geriatrics Society, 56,* 413–420.

Rabins, P. V., Lyketsos, C. G., & Steele, C. D. 2006. *Practical dementia care.* New York: Oxford University Press.

Weiner, M. F., & Lipton, A. M. (Eds.). (2009). *The American Psychiatric Publishing textbook of Alzheimer disease and other dementias.* Arlington, VA: American Psychiatric Publishing.

Zhang, B., Mitchell, S. L., Bambauer, K. Z., et al. (2008). Depressive symptom trajectories and associated risks among bereaved Alzheimer disease caregivers. *American Journal of Geriatric Psychiatry, 16,* 145–155.

SELECTED READINGS FOR THE ALZHEIMER'S FAMILY

Abramson, A. (2004). *The caregiver's survival handbook: How to care for your aging parent without losing yourself.* New York: Perigee.

Bayley, J. (1999). *Elegy for Iris.* New York: Picador.

Bell, V., & Troxel, D. (2002). *A dignified life: The best friends approach to Alzheimer's care. A guide for family caregivers.* Baltimore, MD: Health Professions Press.

Braff, S., & Olenik, M. R. (2003). *Staying connected while letting go: The paradox of Alzheimer's caregiving.* New York: M. Evans.

Buse, F. (2010). *A caregiver's tips: My wife had Alzheimer's disease.* Pittsburgh: Rose Dog Books.

Cade, E. (2002). *Taking care of parents who didn't take care of you: Making peace with aging parents.* Garden City, MN: Hazelden.

Callone, P., Vasiloff, B., Brumback, R., et al. (2005). *A caregiver's guide to Alzheimer's disease: 300 tips for making life easier.* New York: Demos Medical Publishing.

Calo-Oy, S., & Calo-Oy, B. (2004). *The caring caregivers guide to dealing with guilt.* San Antonio, TX: Orchard.

Davidson, A. (2006). *A curious kind of widow: Loving a man with advanced Alzheimer's.* McKinleyville, CA: Fithian Press.

Federico, M. (2009). *Welcome to the Departure Lounge: Adventures in Mothering Mother.* New York: Random House.

Fostino, M. (2007). *Alzheimer's: A caretaker's journal.* New York: Seaboard Press.

Fox, J. (2009). *I still do: Loving and living with Alzheimer's.* New York: Powerhouse Books.

Glenner, J. A., Stehman, J. M., Davagning, J., et al. (2005). *When your loved one has dementia: A simple guide for caregivers.* Baltimore: Johns Hopkins University Press.

Hill, A. P. (2007). *Unforgettable journey: Tips to survive your parent's Alzheimer's disease.* iUniverse.

Koenig-Coste, J. (2003). *Learning to speak Alzheimer's.* Boston: Houghton Mifflin.

Kuster, A. M., with McLane, S. (2004). *The last dance: Facing Alzheimer's with love and laughter.* Portsmouth, NH: Peter E. Randall.

Lebow, G., Kane, B., & Lebow, I. (2000). *Coping with your difficult older parent: A guide for stressed-out children.* New York: Harper.

Mace, N. L., & Rabins, P. V. (1999). *The 36-hour day: A family guide to caring for persons with Alzheimer's disease, related dementing illnesses, and memory loss in later life* (3rd ed.). Baltimore: Johns Hopkins University Press.

McCurry, S. M. (2006). *When a family member has dementia: Steps to becoming a resilient caregiver.* Westport, CT: Praeger.

Montgomery, M. (2010). *Alzheimer Diary: A Wife's Journal.* Charleston, SC: CreateSpace.

Pursley, B. (2009). *Embracing the moment: An Alzheimer's memoir.* Charleston, SC: BookSurge.

Steinberg, R. D. (2010). *Forgetting the memories: A caregiver's journey through Alzheimer's disease.* Bloomington, IN: Authorhouse.

Strauss, C. J. (2001). *Talking to Alzheimer's: Simple ways to connect when you visit with a family member or friend.* Oakland, CA: New Harbinger.

Whybrow, R. (1996). *Caring for elderly parents.* New York: Crossroad.

INTERNET RESOURCES

Alzheimer Research Forum, http://www.alzforum.org/

Alzheimer's Association, http://www.alz.org

Alzheimer's Disease Education and Referral Center (ADEAR), http://www.alzheimers.org/

Alzheimer's Foundation of America (AFA), http://www.alzfdn.org

Caring.com, http://www.caring.com/

Caring Connections, National Hospice and Palliative Care Organization, http:// www.caringinfo.org

Caring from a Distance, http://www.cfad.org/

Eldercare Locator, http://www.eldercare.gov/Eldercare.NET/Public/Index.aspx

Family Caregiver Alliance, http://www.caregiver.org

MedlinePlus Health Information on Alzheimer's Disease, National Library of Medicine, http://www.nlm.nih.gov/medlineplus/alzheimersdisease.html

National Alliance for Caregiving, http://www.caregiving.org/

National Family Caregivers Association, http://www.thefamilycaregiver.org

National Institute on Aging, Alzheimer's Disease Education and Referral Center, http://www.alzheimers.org/index.html

INDEX

management of, 158–59
medications for, 214–15
SNRIs. *see* serotonin-norepinephrine reuptake inhibitors
(SNRIs)
socially inappropriate behaviors,
handling of, 154–55
"someone is stealing my things,"
145
"someone is trying to harm me,"
146
speak slowly, 96
spouse, maintaining physical intimacy with, 107–8
SSRIs. *see* selective serotonin
reuptake inhibitors (SSRIs)
stage(s)
of Alzheimer's disease, 52–55
end, 55, 186–95. *see also* end
stage
late moderate, 170–71
mild, 53–54
moderate, 54–55
severe, 55
statement(s), simple, concrete,
96–97
statins, for cognitive and functional
symptoms of Alzheimer's disease, 204
stigma, of Alzheimer's disease,
56–59
stress, caregiver-related, 161–69.
see also caregiver(s)
stressor(s), memory effects of,
23–24
strong reactions, decreased comprehension of immediate environment leading to, 131
suicide, depression and, 148–149
sundowning
defined, 159

management of, 159–60, 215
support group, 87–88
after death of Alzheimer's patient, 193

"the Alzheimer's family," 2–3,
8–20
"the dementia family," 3
*The Shriver Report: A Woman's
Nation Takes on Alzheimer's,*
2
The 36-Hour Day, 50, 132, 163
thinking, medications affecting,
25–28
"this place is not my house," 147
toileting behaviors, changes in,
42–43
tone of voice, 98
trazodone
for aggressiveness, 210
for anxiety, 212
for sundowning, 215

underlying personality, effects of,
133–34

vascular dementia, 31–35
antidementia medications for,
205–6
vascular disease, dementia due to,
31–35
verbal abuse, by caregiver, 167
vitamin B, for cognitive and functional symptoms of Alzheimer's disease, 204
vitamin C, for cognitive and functional symptoms of Alzheimer's disease, 204
vitamin E, for cognitive and functional symptoms of Alzheimer's disease, 204

DATE DUE

5-20-16		

Demco